Contents

About the editors

Dr Margaret Rees is a Medical Gynaecologist and Reader in Reproductive Medicine in the Nuffield Department of Obstetrics and Gynaecology, University of Oxford. She runs the menopause clinic in Oxford – one of the first founded in the UK. She is Editor-in-Chief of the *Journal of the British Menopause Society*, and an expert advisor to Women's Health Concern.

Professor David Purdie is Consultant to the Edinburgh Osteoporosis Centre and has a long clinical and research interest in the detection and treatment of osteoporosis. He is a former Chairman of Council of the British Menopause Society and a member of the scientific advisory group of the National Osteoporosis Society.

Dr Sally Hope is a General Practitioner in Woodstock, Oxfordshire. She has developed a special interest in women's health over the past 20 years. She is an Honorary Lecturer in the Department of Primary Care, University of Oxford. She is a founder member of the Primary Care Group in Gynaecology, and served on the Council of the British Menopause Society for three years. She is a deputy editor of the *Journal of the British Menopause Society*.

The Menopause: What you need to know

2nd edition

Editors

D???? ?urdie and S???

BRITISH MENOPAUSE SOCIETY
Meeting the Challenge of Menopause

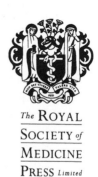

The ROYAL
SOCIETY of
MEDICINE
PRESS Limited

© 2006 Royal Society of Medicine Press Ltd and British Menopause Society Publications Ltd

Published by the Royal Society of Medicine Press Ltd   *and*   British Menopause Society Publications Ltd
1 Wimpole Street, London W1G 0AE, UK
Tel: +44 (0)20 7290 2921
Fax: +44 (0)20 7290 2929
Email: publishing@rsm.ac.uk
Website: www.rsmpress.co.uk

4–6 Eton Place, Marlow SL7 2QA, UK
Tel: +44 (0)1628 890199
Fax: +44 (0)1628 474024
Email: admin.bms@btconnect.com
Website: www.the-bms.org

British Menopause Society (registered charity no. 10151440)

British Library Cataloguing in Publication Data
A catalogue record for this book is available from the British Library
ISBN 1-85315-672-8

Distribution in Europe and Rest of World:
Marston Book Services Ltd
PO Box 269
Abingdon
Oxon OX14 4YN, UK
Tel: +44 (0)1235 465500
Fax: +44 (0)1235 465555
Email: direct.order@marston.co.uk

Distribution in the USA and Canada:
Royal Society of Medicine Press Ltd
c/o BookMasters, Inc.
30 Amberwood Parkway
Ashland, Ohio 44805, USA
Tel: +1 800 247 6553 / +1 800 266 5564
Email: order@bookmasters.com

Distribution in Australia and New Zealand:
Elsevier Australia
30–52 Smidmore Street
Marrickville NSW 2204
Australia
Tel: + 61 2 9349 5811
Fax: + 61 2 9349 5911
Email: service@elsevier.com.au

Designed and typeset by Phoenix Photosetting, Chatham, Kent
Printed and bound by Krips b.v., Meppel, The Netherlands

Preface

All women will go through the menopause and the average age at which this happens is 52 years. Women and health professionals are divided over how to approach the menopause. Some feel it is a natural event that should not normally need medical treatment. Others believe that the effects that occur after the ovaries stop producing hormones represent an important medical condition.

Whatever our beliefs, however, there is no doubt that although some women have no problems, others experience considerable stress around the time that their monthly periods end. Evidence also shows that the change in hormone production can lead to conditions such as thinning bones. This can have a major effect on the quality of many women's lives.

One problem in understanding the menopause is that it is a relatively new experience. Until the 19th century, most women simply did not live long enough to reach the menopause, and doctors only started studying it about 60 years ago.

The aim of this book is to provide unbiased and non-promotional information about managing the menopause. The ultimate decision about what course to take needs to be made after talking to a health professional. The book is based on the *British Menopause Society Handbook*, which was written by menopause specialists for family doctors, gynaecologists, nurses and other health professionals. The first edition was produced in 1994, and it was last updated in January 2006. Its success prompted the British Menopause Society to bring out this version for the people who actually have to face the menopause and its consequences. Where possible, we have avoided using medical language, but we have included definitions of words that health professionals might use. The word list at the end of the book gives definitions of these terms, and they are shown in *italics* when they are first used in each chapter. In the sections entitled 'Sources of information' at the end of each chapter, you will find a series of journal, book and website references. These are not exhaustive lists but aim to show what is available. The journals are listed on Medline and can be accessed through the following website: www.ncbi.nlm.nih.gov/entrez/query.fcgi. Website addresses may change from time to time, but they should be found by searching for the name of the organization.

The British Menopause Society (a registered charity) was founded in 1989 as an independent scientific society for health professionals. Its aims are to raise awareness about the menopause and improve the treatment that menopausal women receive. It organizes clinical and scientific meetings and produces a scientific journal for healthcare professionals

Dr Margaret Rees
Professor David W Purdie
Dr Sally Hope
June 2006

Acknowledgements

We thank the council members of the British Menopause Society and other medical experts who contributed to the doctors' handbook and to this version, as well as Dr Barbara Burge (general practitioner), Melbourne, Australia and Associate Professor Cornelia Amalinei, Iasi, Romania. We also thank the following non-medical people who reviewed this second edition of the book and gave us helpful comments:

- Ray Anson, Oxford
- Josie Ferguson, Oxford
- Susan Foley, Wellington, New Zealand
- Christine Gillson, Oxford
- Robert Gillson, Oxford
- Rita Lockwood, Haddenham
- Dee Nudds, Oxford
- Charles Sowerwine, Melbourne, Australia
- Anneli Stavreus-Evers, Stockholm, Sweden

Liz Wager of Sideview reworked the text of the doctors' handbook to produce this version.

1 What is the menopause?

The menopause is the time when a woman's monthly periods finally stop. The word menopause comes from the Greek words *menos*, meaning a month, and *pausos*, which means an ending. As it is not always possible to define the point at which periods stop, doctors have agreed the following definitions.

Definitions

Menopause

Because menopause means the final monthly period, it can be recognized only after the event. In medical terms, the menopause is considered to have occurred after a woman has gone for 12 months without having periods, as long as there is no other reason for this. If a woman is still having periods, even if they are irregular, the menopause has not yet occurred. Although your doctor may take a blood test to measure hormone levels, no single measurement can confirm that the menopause has occurred.

Premenopause

The term premenopause can be used to mean the period just one or two years before the menopause or the whole of a woman's reproductive life before the menopause. In this book, we use it to mean the entire phase from a woman's first monthly period to her last.

Perimenopause

Perimenopause describes the time from when a woman first notices menopausal symptoms, such as hot flushes or irregular periods, until 12 months after her last monthly period.

Postmenopause

Postmenopause means the time after a woman's last menstrual period. For women whose menopause is caused by *oophorectomy* (an operation to remove the ovaries), the start of the postmenopause may be obvious. For those who have a natural menopause, it cannot be determined until they have had 12 months without periods.

Menopause transition

The menopause transition is the time just before the final menstrual period. Many women have irregular periods during this phase. The length of the menopause transition varies from woman to woman and may last several years.

Climacteric

This term refers to a woman's transition from the reproductive to the non-reproductive state. Strictly speaking, the menopause is just one event that occurs during the climacteric, just as *menarche* (when monthly periods start) is just one event in puberty.

Climacteric syndrome

Many, but not all, women experience symptoms around the menopause. The collection of symptoms is sometimes referred to as the climacteric syndrome.

Premature or early menopause

The average age when most women's periods stop is about 52 years. This is considered a normal menopause, but there is considerable variation either side of this and between women in different countries. In addition, estimates of the average age at menopause in developing countries may not always be accurate. It therefore is quite difficult to define a premature menopause. The age of 40 years is used frequently as an arbitrary limit below which the menopause is said to be premature. In developed countries such as the UK, however, menopause occurring before a woman is aged 45 years is considered early. Premature menopause is covered in more detail in Chapter 12.

Induced menopause

This term is used to describe a menopause caused by surgery (such as an oophorectomy), chemotherapy, radiotherapy or other medical treatment. It contrasts with the natural or spontaneous menopause, which would otherwise have occurred when a woman reached the age of about 52 years.

When does the menopause happen?

The timing of the menopause may be determined even before a woman is born or can be affected by events in early childhood. Women who were small as babies or were malnourished as children tend to have an early menopause. Smokers also tend to have an earlier menopause than non-smokers. Genetics may also play a part, as Japanese women usually have a later age of natural menopause than European women.

In the UK, a woman's average life expectancy from birth is 81 years. The average age of menopause is 52 years. British women can therefore expect more than 30 years of life after the menopause. For those women who live to 100 years, the menopause can now be considered a mid-life event!

What causes the menopause?

A woman's monthly menstrual periods stop when her ovaries (the female reproductive organs) stop working or are removed.

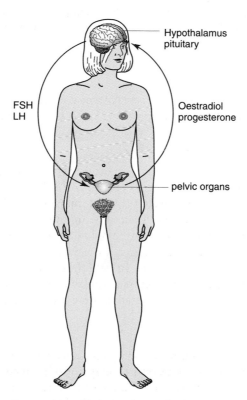

Figure 1.1 Interactions between the hypothalamus, pituitary gland and ovaries

Role of the ovaries

The ovaries are controlled by two hormones that are produced by a small gland called the pituitary gland that lies just underneath the brain (Figure 1.1). These hormones are called follicle-stimulating hormone (*FSH*) and luteinizing hormone (*LH*). They are controlled by another hormone called gonadotrophin-releasing hormone (GnRH), which is produced in the brain itself. Gonadotrophin-releasing hormone in turn is affected by chemicals produced by the ovaries. The ovaries produce the two female hormones oestradiol and *progesterone*, which act on the womb lining (or *endometrium*) to cause periods (Figure 1.2). In premenopausal women, the levels of these sex hormones in the blood change regularly over the course of the monthly menstrual cycle and also regulate the levels of GnRH (Figure 1.3). When the ovaries are functioning, they also secrete a small protein called inhibin; high levels of inhibin stop the secretion of GnRH. When a woman is fertile, her ovaries normally release one egg cell during every cycle – this is known as ovulation.

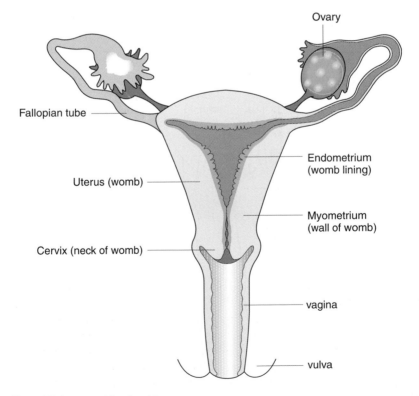

Figure 1.2 Anatomy of female pelvic organs

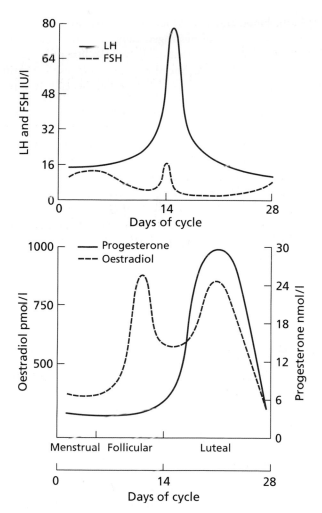

Figure 1.3 Hormone levels during a normal menstrual cycle

The egg cells (or *oocytes*) are laid down in a woman's ovaries before she is born. From that point on the number decreases until, about 50 years later, very few are left. As a woman ages, her ovaries gradually become less responsive to FSH and LH and produce less *oestrogen*. Although the woman may still have monthly bleeds, the number of anovulatory menstrual cycles – during which no egg is released – gradually increases towards the menopause.

Around the menopause, the levels of female sex hormones may fluctuate almost daily, but over time, there is a gradual increase in levels of FSH and then of LH in the blood and a fall in levels of oestradiol and inhibin (Figure 1.4). Consistently low levels of oestrogen cause a woman's periods to stop. Levels of FSH higher than 30 international units per litre of blood are usually a sign that the ovaries are failing and that the menopause is nearing or has occurred. In premenopausal women, FSH levels are usually 10 international units per litre of blood or lower.

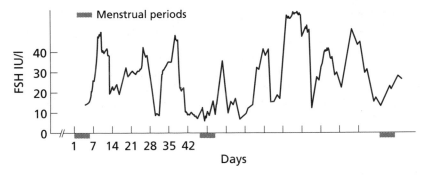

Figure 1.4 Levels of follicle-stimulating hormone during the menopause

Why does the menopause happen?

Women lose their fertility much earlier than other animal species, and some scientists believe that the human menopause evolved to protect women and their children from the dangers of late childbearing. One important difference between us and other mammals is that human children depend on their parents for a longer period of their lives. Our highly evolved brain means that, at birth, human babies have larger heads than other species, which makes childbirth more difficult. Because of this, human babies spend a relatively short time in the womb and therefore are born at a less developed stage than other mammals. The risks of childbirth to both the mother and baby increase as the mother gets older. For older women, there therefore may be little survival advantage in further pregnancies, when her earlier children still depend on her for their survival.

Another explanation is that humans have evolved into extended family groups, and the presence of postmenopausal grandmothers might help their daughters to raise their grandchildren.

However, not all scientists accept these evolutionary explanations. Some believe that the menopause is simply the result of the fact that humans live much longer than other mammals of a similar size. All mammals and birds form their female reproductive cells before birth, so we start life with a limited number of eggs and our ovaries may simply run out of eggs as our bodies age.

Sources of information

Journal articles

Hardy R, Kuh D. Social and environmental conditions across the life course and age at menopause in a British birth cohort study. *BJOG* 2005; **112**: 346–54.

Landgren BM, Collins A, Csemiczky G *et al.* Menopause transition: annual changes in serum hormonal patterns over the menstrual cycle in women during a nine-year period prior to menopause. *J Clin Endocrinol Metab* 2004; **89**: 2763–9.

Lawlor DA, Ebrahim S, Smith GD. The association of socio-economic position across the life course and age at menopause: the British Women's Heart and Health Study. *BJOG* 2003; **110**: 1078–87.

Reynolds RF, Obermeyer CM. Age at natural menopause in Spain and the United States: results from the DAMES project. *Am J Hum Biol* 2005; **17**: 331–40.

Van Asselt KM, Kok HS, van Der Schouw YT *et al.* Current smoking at menopause rather than duration determines the onset of natural menopause. *Epidemiology* 2004; **15**: 634–9.

Websites

MedlinePlus – Women's Health Issues:
www.nlm.nih.gov/medlineplus/womenshealthissues.html (last accessed 5 March 2006).

Menopausematters:
www.menopausematters.co.uk (last accessed 5 March 2006).

Medical Information for Women:
www.gynaeuk.com (last accessed 9 March 2006)

Women's Health Concern:
www.womens-health-concern.org (last accessed 5 March 2006).

2 Symptoms of the menopause

Vasomotor symptoms (hot flushes and night sweats)
Sexual problems
Psychological symptoms
Sources of information

Changes in hormone levels, particularly a fall in the level of *oestrogen*, can cause symptoms around the menopause. Approximately 70% of women experience symptoms such as hot flushes and night sweats. Some women also report psychological symptoms, which may be linked to their other symptoms or may be a reaction to menstrual changes or other life events. These include tiredness, lack of energy, depressed mood, aches and pains, and reduced interest in sex. Cultural differences in women's attitudes to the menopause probably exist: for example, Japanese women report fewer symptoms than American women.

Vasomotor symptoms (hot flushes and night sweats)

Hot flushes and night sweats are the most common symptoms of the menopause and can occur before the periods stop (Figure 2.1). Flushes occur most often in the first year after the last period and are caused by a malfunction in the body's normal methods of controlling its temperature. Women who have hot flushes cannot control body heat normally (the so-called *vasomotor* response) and skin temperature goes up during a hot flush. Hot flushes can occur at any time of the day or night. Night-time flushes and sweats can disturb a woman's sleep patterns, which may lead to insomnia, irritability and difficulties with memory and concentration.

Sexual problems

Changes in sexual behaviour and activity are not uncommon in menopausal women. Both men and women gradually lose interest in sex as they get older, but the decrease seems to be more marked in women. Older women may

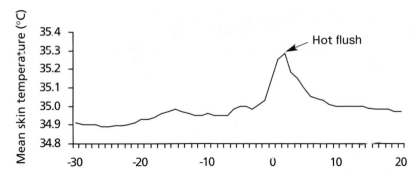

Figure 2.1 Mean skin temperature during hot flushes. Adapted from Freedman RR (1998), with permission from American Society for Reproductive Medicine

experience less desire for sex (loss of *libido*), may find it harder to become sexually aroused or to have an orgasm and may find sex painful. These problems may be caused by several different factors and are sometimes termed female sexual dysfunction (FSD). There is now a classification of sexual problems to help treatment and research. The four categories are:

- lack of desire
- lack of arousal
- problems with orgasm
- painful sex.

Lower levels of oestrogen cause vaginal dryness, which may make sex uncomfortable. Painful intercourse may reduce the desire for sex, and anticipation of discomfort can cause lack of arousal. Hormone levels may also affect a woman's sensory perception. Interest in sex may also decrease if a woman's sleep is disturbed by night sweats and hot flushes or if she feels depressed. Menopausal symptoms may also contribute to difficulties in relationships, which makes matters worse. But the problems may not always lie with the woman, and male sexual problems, such as loss of libido and erection problems, should not be overlooked.

Psychological symptoms

Psychological symptoms, including depressed mood, anxiety, irritability, mood swings, tiredness and lack of energy, have been linked to the menopause. However, large population surveys suggest that most women do not have major mood changes around their menopause. The psychological problems reported during the menopause are more likely to be associated with past problems and with stressful events that happen to occur around this stage of a woman's life such as:

- parents' ageing and becoming less independent
- death of parents, relatives or friends
- loss of a partner through death, separation or divorce
- lack of social support
- children leaving home or 'empty nest syndrome'
- worries over children's education, jobs or relationships
- poor health
- demanding workload or job insecurity
- money problems
- coming to terms with ageing in a culture that values youth and fertility.

These factors, together with the physical changes of the menopause, can combine to make a woman feel stressed and unable to cope. Because the factors are different for every woman, you have to make your own choice about what you do about them and whether or not you seek medical treatment. Lack of sleep caused by night sweats can cause psychological symptoms, so treatments that reduce these vasomotor symptoms may be helpful in reducing other symptoms.

Sources of information

Journal articles

Basson R, Berman J, Burnett A *et al.* Report of the international consensus development conference on female sexual dysfunction: definitions and classifications. *J Urol* 2000; **163**: 888–93.

Cohen LS, Soares CN, Joffe H. Diagnosis and management of mood disorders during the menopausal transition. *Am J Med* 2005; **118** (12 Suppl 2): 93–7.

Dennerstein L, Guthrie JR, Clark M *et al.* A population-based study of depressed mood in middle-aged, Australian-born women. *Menopause* 2004; **11**: 563–8.

Freedman RR. Biochemical, metabolic, and vascular mechanisms in menopausal hot flashes. *Fertil Steril* 1998; **70**(2): 332–7

Li C, Samsioe G, Borgfeldt C *et al.* Menopause-related symptoms: what are the background factors? A prospective population-based cohort study of Swedish women (The Women's Health in Lund Area study). *Am J Obstet Gynecol* 2003; **189**: 1646–53.

Lock M. Symptom reporting at menopause: a review of cross-cultural findings. *J Br Menopause Soc* 2002; **8**: 132–6.

Morley JE, Kaiser FE. Female sexuality. *Med Clin North Am* 2003; **87**: 1077–90.

Book

Tomlinson JM, Rees M, Mander T, eds. *Sexual Health and the Menopause.* London: Royal Society of Medicine Press, 2005.

Websites

Sexual Health Network:
   www.sexualhealth.com (last accessed 6 March 2006).
Sexual Health UK:
   www.sexualhealthuk.info

3 Long-term effects of the menopause

The ageing population
Osteoporosis (brittle bones)
Cardiovascular disease
Dementia
Urinary problems
Sources of information

The long-term effects of the menopause probably affect the quality, and even the length, of women's lives more than the short-term symptoms. However, these effects may be hard to measure, as they often remain clinically silent for many years.

The ageing population

Increasing life expectancy means that the number of people older than 65 years is projected to grow considerably worldwide. In 2002, 440 million people were older than 65 years; this was about 7% of the total population. This figure is projected to increase rapidly, and it is estimated that elderly people will comprise nearly 17% of the world's population in 2050. The percentage of elderly people is high in the countries that make up the developed world and very low in Africa and the Near East.

In the UK, the population is projected to increase by 7.2 million over the period 2004–31 and will continue to rise thereafter (Figure 3.1). Life expectancy at birth will continue to rise from 81 years to 85 years in women and 76 years to 81 years in men. The population expansion will lead to an increasing importance of the health problems that affect postmenopausal women.

Osteoporosis (brittle bones)

As men and women get older, their bones become weaker (Figure 3.2). This is called *osteoporosis*. Bone strength depends on the density of the bone tissue

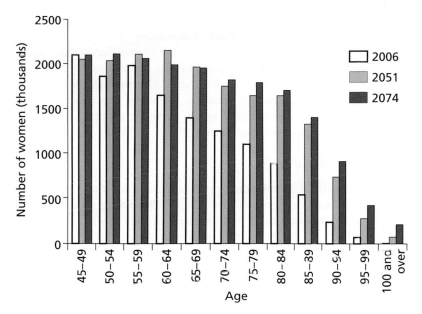

Figure 3.1 Population projections for the UK. Adapted from the Office of National Statistics and Government Actuaries Department (2005)

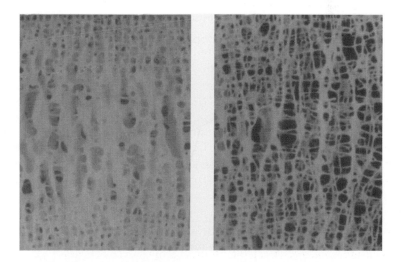

Figure 3.2 Normal (left) and osteoporotic (right) bone in the spine

and its structure. Reduced amounts of minerals in the bone and slower production or replacement of bone cells can weaken the bones. Although everybody's bones get weaker as they get older, the change occurs much faster in women after the menopause. This explains why one in three women have osteoporosis compared with only one in 12 men. Osteoporosis increases the risk of breaking bones, especially those in the wrist, hip or spine. Such fractures can have a major effect on a person's quality of life and independence…and may even shorten their life.

Bone mineral density

The density (heaviness) of bones can be measured, and this can show whether or not a person has osteoporosis (see Chapter 5). Severe osteoporosis is recognized when a person has a bone mineral density reading (called a T score) lower than –2.5. At this stage, they are also likely to get bone fractures from minor accidents that would not cause fractures in people with stronger bones, such as falling from a chair.

Bone mineral density and age

Bone density increases during the teenage years and reaches a peak sometime in the mid-20s (Figure 3.3). This peak bone density is sustained for some years, but the density starts to decline during the mid-40s. For 6–10 years after the menopause, women lose bone rapidly. After that, bone loss continues but at a much slower rate. Once bone reaches a certain stage, even a minor injury will cause it to break.

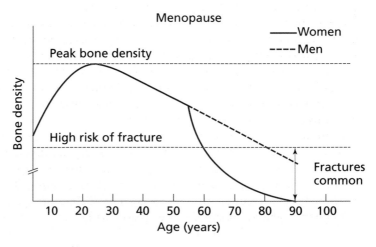

Figure 3.3 Patterns of bone loss with age

Three factors determine whether or not a woman develops osteoporosis. These are:

- how strong her bones were when she was in her 20s (her peak bone mass)
- how fast her bones thin after the menopause
- and how long she lives after the menopause.

Men generally develop osteoporosis much later than women, because they have a much higher peak bone mass and do not suffer the rapid loss that occurs after the menopause.

Men do not have the equivalent of the female menopause, in which there is a sudden fall in hormone levels – levels of *testosterone* gradually decline with age in men.

Factors that probably increase peak bone mass are:

- a diet high in calcium and vitamin D
- not smoking (especially in your teenage years)
- taking weight-bearing exercise (such as jogging).

However, there have been no trials in teenagers to confirm that these really do prevent osteoporosis in later life.

Risk factors for osteoporosis
Risk of osteoporosis varies among ethnic groups, and white people suffer more fractures than those of African–Caribbean origin. Osteoporosis is probably not caused by a single gene, but a woman's risk of developing it may be the result of variations in several genes. Bone density is largely determined by inherited factors, with lifestyle factors playing a lesser role.

The injectable depot contraceptive Depo-Provera (sometimes called DPMA or depot *medroxyprogesterone acetate*) probably causes a small amount of bone loss (5–10%), but this does not increase over time. Healthy women of normal build who have a good diet and lifestyle need not worry about this. Women with a family history of osteoporosis and a personal history of smoking, poor diet or little exercise should discuss this with their doctor, who may suggest a bone scan or recommend another type of contraception.

Certain groups of women have a high risk of a fracture because of osteoporosis (see Chapter 6). However, it is not always easy to assess the risk for an individual woman, because the effects of some factors are small. The most important factors seem to be family history (for example, if your mother has had a hip fracture), an early menopause (before the age of 45 years), long-term *glucocorticosteroid* use (particularly tablets such as prednisolone but possibly also the use of steroids in asthma inhalers), long-term immobility and previous fractures.

Effects of osteoporosis

The main consequence of osteoporosis is broken bones. The bones that most often get broken are those in the wrist, hip and spine (back and neck). Falling on an outstretched hand often causes *Colles' fractures* of the radius bone in the wrist, which are painful and severely limit the use of the arm and hand.

Hip fractures in young women are unusual and are most commonly caused by road accidents. However, in older women with brittle bones, hips can be broken by falls or may even fracture spontaneously. Women are twice as likely to have a hip fracture than men. One in seven British women (14%) break a hip sometime after their menopause. Broken hips cause more deaths, disability and medical costs than all of the other osteoporotic fractures combined. A woman who has broken her hip is more likely to die the following year than if she had not broken it. One in two patients with a broken hip will have some permanent disability or loss of independence.

The effects of osteoporosis on the spine (vertebral fractures) are hard to measure, because there are often no symptoms until the spine has become seriously deformed (Figure 3.4). Vertebral fractures often cause general back

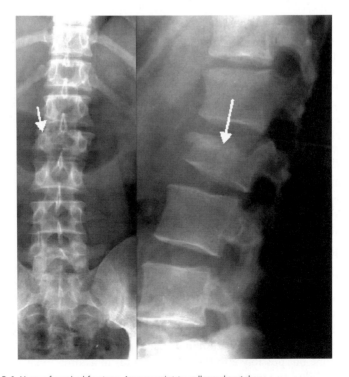

Figure 3.4 X-ray of a spinal fracture. Arrows point to collapsed vertebra

pain, and up to 90% are never seen by doctors. Multiple fractures cause height loss and a characteristic stooping (the so-called 'dowager's hump'). They can cause considerable pain and loss of quality of life and may eventually restrict breathing. Presence of one vertebral fracture suggests a high risk of future fractures – both in the spine and elsewhere.

The main goal of research into osteoporosis is to prevent the first fracture and to identify women at particular risk.

Cardiovascular disease

Cardiovascular disease means any disease of the heart or blood vessels. The major diseases in this group are heart attacks and strokes and are usually caused by blocked arteries. Although cardiovascular disease rarely kills women younger than 60 years, it is the most common cause of death in older women (Figure 3.5). Heart disease and stroke together account for about one-third of deaths. Some evidence (mainly from animal studies) shows that women are more likely to suffer from blocked arteries after the menopause. Studies of women who have had an operation to remove their ovaries (*oophorectomy*) suggest that they are 2–3 times more likely to have a *coronary* (heart attack) than women of the same age who still have their ovaries and are premenopausal.

Coronary heart disease

Coronary heart disease (*CHD*) is the biggest single cause of death in British women. Although it accounts for about one in four of all female deaths, CHD is still often considered, wrongly, to be largely a male problem. The rate of

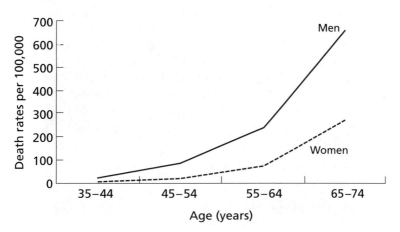

Figure 3.5 Rates of heart disease in men and women. Source: Department of Health (2003)

CHD increases after the menopause, but the rate of increase is remarkably similar in men and women older than 50 years. Some studies have suggested that women have more problems such as angina and palpitations after a heart attack than men, but men are far more likely to suffer another, this time fatal, heart attack. The death rate from treatments such as heart bypass operations seems to be higher for women than men.

A heart attack (or *myocardial infarction*) happens when one or more of the major (coronary) arteries supplying the heart muscle with blood become blocked. This starves the heart muscle of oxygen, so that it cannot pump properly. Arteries usually become blocked because a blood clot (or *thrombus*) forms in a vessel that has been narrowed by a build-up of fatty material called a plaque. Such narrowing of the arteries is called *atherosclerosis*.

Stroke

The rate of strokes increases with age. One in five 50-year-old white British women will have a stroke during their lifetime. Strokes kill large numbers of women and leave many others with serious disabilities. A stroke happens when part of the brain is starved of oxygen. The most common cause of stroke is a blood clot blocking an *artery* that supplies blood to the brain. Strokes can also be caused by bleeding (*haemorrhage*) in the brain.

Dementia

This term is used to describe conditions in which patients lose their memory and cannot think clearly. *Dementia* can also cause psychological problems and behavioural changes. Common forms of dementia include Alzheimer's disease, vascular dementia and Lewy body dementia. Symptoms of dementia can cause great stress to patients, their carers and families. Women have a central role in caring for people with dementia. It has been estimated that 24.3 million people throughout the world have dementia today, with 4.6 million new cases of dementia every year (one new case every seven seconds). The number of people affected will double every 20 years to 81.1 million by 2040. There are a number of new drug treatments (such as *donepezil, galantamine, memantine* and *rivastigmine*) that may help.

Urinary problems

Low *oestrogen* levels can affect the bladder and the muscles that control it. This may cause symptoms such as:

- increased urinary frequency (needing to pass water often)
- the need to pass water at night (*nocturia*)
- urgency

- incontinence
- recurring infections

The changes in the bladder are similar to those that occur in the vagina and cause dryness and discomfort (see the section in Chapter 2 on sexual problems). Therefore these changes are sometimes called urogenital atrophy. Urinary incontinence is mortifying for women. Specialist clinics can identify specific problems in the bladder that may be helped by medicines (such as *darifenacin, duloxetine, oxybutynin, solfenacin, tolterodine* and *trospium*) or surgery.

Sources of information

Journal articles

Cooper C, Westlake S, Harvey N *et al.* Review: developmental origins of osteoporotic fracture. *Osteoporos Int* 2006; **17**: 337–47.

Ferri CP, Prince M, Brayne C *et al.* Global prevalence of dementia: a Delphi consensus study. *Lancet* 2005; **366**: 2112–17.

Lansky AJ, Pietras C, Costa RA *et al.* Gender differences in outcomes after primary angioplasty versus primary stenting with and without abciximab for acute myocardial infarction: results of the Controlled Abciximab and Device Investigation to Lower Late Angioplasty Complications (CADILLAC) trial. *Circulation* 2005; **111**: 1611–18.

McGrother CW, Donaldson MM, Hayward T *et al.* Urinary storage symptoms and comorbidities: a prospective population cohort study in middle-aged and older women. *Age Ageing* 2006; **35**: 16–24.

Strong K, Mathers C, Leeder S, Beaglehole R. Preventing chronic diseases: how many lives can we save? *Lancet* 2005; **366**: 1578–82.

Book

Keith LG, Rees M, Mander T, eds. *Menopause, Postmenopause and Ageing.* London: Royal Society of Medicine Press, 2005.

Websites

Alzheimer's Society:
www.alzheimers.org.uk (last accessed 6 March 2006).
British Heart Foundation (BHF):
www.bhf.org.uk (last accessed 6 March 2006).
Government Actuary's Department (GAD):
www.gad.gov.uk (last accessed 6 March 2006).
Incontact (organization in the UK for people affected by bladder and bowel problems):
www.incontact.org (last accessed 6 March 2006).
National Osteoporosis Society:
www.nos.org.uk (last accessed 6 March 2006).

4 Contraception and sexual health

Contraception around the menopause

You should not assume that you cannot get pregnant just because you have some signs of the menopause or are using hormone replacement therapy (*HRT*). You should continue to use contraception for two years after your last period if you are younger than 50 years and for at least one year if you are older than 50 years. There are reliable reports of women who have given birth in their 50s. The oldest woman known to have had a baby without *in vitro* fertilization was 57 years old.

Your preferred method of contraceptive may change around the menopause, so information about different methods is presented below.

Natural family planning

These methods are not reliable around the menopause. At this time, your cycle becomes unpredictable, temperature changes are inconsistent and the nature of the cervical mucus changes. Methods that rely on measuring hormone levels at ovulation also become unreliable. To avoid pregnancy, therefore, you should use another method of contraception

Coitus interruptus (withdrawal)

This method is unreliable, but it may be the method of choice if you have used it successfully before. Vaginal dryness, fear of pregnancy and changes in your *libido* or your partner's libido or potency may make it more difficult.

Condoms

You can continue to use condoms, but you may find that they make sex uncomfortable. Dryness of the vagina also means that condoms are more likely to split. You should therefore use lubricating or spermicidal gels. Remember that some vaginal preparations such as *oestrogen* creams and pessaries can weaken condoms and make them more likely to split.

Diaphragm (cap)

You can continue to use a diaphragm (cap), but changes in the vagina may make it difficult to fit or keep in place. Remember that some vaginal preparations such as oestrogen creams and pessaries can affect the rubber used in diaphragms and make them unreliable.

Spermicides

These may make sex more comfortable by increasing lubrication and are more effective in older women than younger women. Spermicides can be used alone (such as a foam or pessary) or with a barrier method (such as a diaphragm). Changes to the vagina at the menopause can make you more sensitive to the chemicals in spermicides, so there is more risk of irritation or allergy.

Intrauterine devices (IUDs or coils)

If you already have an intrauterine device fitted, you can continue to rely on it for contraception. It can be left in place until you no longer need contraception. Use of an IUD may increase the chance of abnormal bleeding.

Intrauterine systems (IUS)

Intrauterine devices that release *progestogen* offer effective contraception and can also be used in combination with the effects of oestrogen in HRT (Figure 4.1). They can therefore be used to provide bleed-free HRT for women going through the menopause.

Combined oral contraceptives (the pill)

Low-dose pills provide reliable contraception, as well as the benefits of oestrogen replacement in older women. Women who do not smoke, have normal blood pressure, are not overweight and do not have a family history of blood clots or breast cancer can continue using these pills until at least their mid-40s or early 50s. However, they may cause a slightly increased risk of breast cancer and possibly also heart attacks and strokes.

Progestogen only pills (mini-pill)

These are suitable for use throughout the perimenopause, and there is no upper age limit for their use. In fact, the effectiveness of the mini-pill

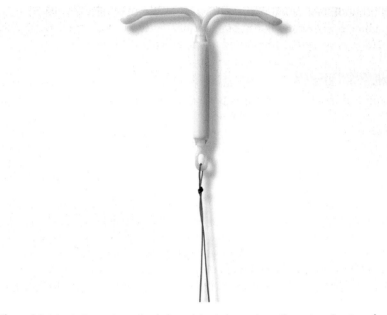

Figure 4.1 Intrauterine contraceptive device or intrauterine contraceptive system. Courtesy of Schering Health Care, UK

improves as women get older. Not much information is available about the effects of using the mini-pill in combination with HRT.

Implants (intramuscular and subdermal progestogens)

If you have an injected or implanted contraceptive (Figure 4.2), lack of periods can make it hard to tell when the menopause takes place, but they provide reliable contraception and are suitable for use during the menopause. Not much information is available about the effects of using them in combination with HRT.

Sterilization (male or female)

Sterilization (vasectomy for men and clipping the Fallopian tubes for women) is the most common form of pregnancy prevention in older couples in the UK. It is reliable and has no effect on treatments for the menopause.

Sexual health

Going through the menopause does not mean that you can ignore your sexual health and abandon safe sex. The rate of HIV/AIDS in people older than 50 years is rising rapidly, especially among heterosexual people. In the UK, rates

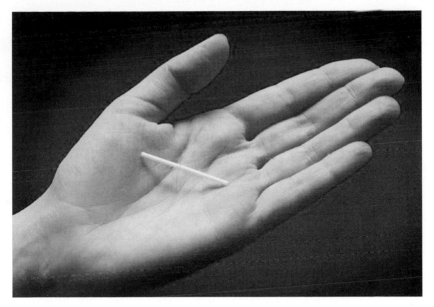

Figure 4.2 Implanted contraceptive device. Courtesy of Organon, UK

of other sexually transmitted infections (STIs) such as syphilis and gonorrhoea have also risen sharply in women aged 45–64 years since the mid 1990s. Even when you no longer need contraception, you still need to protect yourself against STIs.

Sources of information

Journal articles

Faculty of Family Planning and Reproductive Health Care Clinical Effectiveness Unit. Contraception for women aged over 40 years. *J Fam Plann Reprod Health Care* 2005; **31**: 51–64.

Peterson HB, Curtis KM. Clinical practice. Long-acting methods of contraception. *N Engl J Med* 2005; **353**: 2169–75.

Ward DJ, Rowe B, Pattison H *et al.* Reducing the risk of sexually transmitted infections in genitourinary medicine clinic patients: a systematic review and meta-analysis of behavioural interventions. *Sex Transm Infect* 2005; **81**: 386–93.

Websites

Family Planning Association:
www.fpa.org.uk (last accessed 6 March 2006).
Health Protection Agency:
www.hpa.org.uk (last accessed 6 March 2006).

5 What you need to know about tests

Hormone tests
Examining the womb and its lining (endometrium)
Tests for osteoporosis
Genetic testing
Routine tests for all women
Sources of information

Your doctor might suggest that you have some tests to check your:

- hormone levels
- womb, if you have unexpected vaginal bleeding
- bones.

You should discuss any tests with your doctor and ask for the results to be explained to you.

Hormone tests

Sometimes, problems that occur around the menopause have nothing to do with *oestrogen* levels, so it is important to rule out other conditions (Table 5.1). Your doctor might order blood or urine tests if they suspect this might be the case or if you have menopausal symptoms that are not responding to hormone replacement therapy (*HRT*).

Testosterone levels

Both men and women produce the hormone *testosterone* (although men produce much higher amounts than women). This may be linked with levels of sexual appetite (*libido*). However, nearly all the testosterone in the blood is bound to other chemicals, so it does not show up on tests. Therefore, simple measures of the amount of testosterone in the blood are not particularly helpful.

Table 5.1

Tests to rule out other conditions in women with menopausal symptoms

Test	Reason for test
Follicle-stimulating hormone (FSH) levels in blood	This is usually done in women younger than 45 years if their doctor is unsure whether or not the menopause has started or if the ovaries are not working properly
Oestradiol in blood	To see how well the woman is absorbing or responding to oestradiol, such as from an implant, patch or gel
Thyroid function in blood	To rule out thyroid problems, which are easily confused with menopausal symptoms
Catecholamines or 5-hydroxyindolacetic acid in urine	To exclude very rare causes of hot flushes (phaeochromocytoma and carcinoid syndrome)

Examining the womb and its lining (endometrium)

Taking HRT alters a woman's risk of problems in the womb lining (*endometrium*) (see Chapter 8). Various tests can be performed: these are described below.

Ultrasound scans

The first test is usually a scan. This is usually done in your vagina but can also be done through your tummy wall. It will look at the womb and the ovaries. It will look not only at the endometrium but will also check for *fibroids* or cysts on your ovaries.

Biopsy

A *biopsy* or small sample of tissue may need to be taken from the lining of the womb. A biopsy is usually done without an anaesthetic by passing a fine tube through the neck of the womb and obtaining the tissue with gentle suction. The procedure is similar to having a smear. You may have some period-like pain during and after the procedure. In some cases, however, the biopsy is obtained under general anaesthetic – usually as a day-case procedure – and has been called a dilatation and curettage (D&C).

Hysteroscopy

A *hysteroscopy* gives direct viewing of the inside of the womb. It involves passing a fine telescope inside the womb through the neck of the womb and can be done without or with a general anaesthetic.

Tests for osteoporosis

Scans to test the density of bone are not recommended for healthy women. However, they can be useful for women at high risk of *osteoporosis* or who are already thought to have brittle bones (see Chapters 3, 6 and 9).

Scans using X-rays

Scans generally use X-rays at two different energies to separate and identify soft tissue and bone. The process may therefore be called *dual-energy X-ray absorptiometry* (DXA). This can accurately measure the mineral density of the bone (Figure 5.1). This technique is considered to be the 'gold-standard' method and measures density in the hip and the spine. In order to reduce the risks of repeated X-rays, bone scans are usually repeated only after about three years, although a second scan may be given 1–2 years after a new treatment has been started to measure its effects. *Single-energy X-ray absorptiometry* is commonly used for wrist scans; it is not as accurate as hip and spine measurements.

Scans using ultrasound

Ultrasound systems are also being developed to measure bone strength in the heel. The machines used have the advantage of being portable and not using

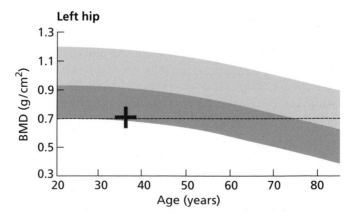

Figure 5.1 Bone density in part of the hip in a healthy population

X-rays; however, they need further testing before they are used more widely. Their main role is to help identify women at high risk of osteoporosis rather than diagnosing the condition or following up women on treatment.

Blood or urine tests

In future, it may also be possible to diagnose osteoporosis from a blood or urine test, by looking at chemicals associated with bone build up or breakdown. Such a test should be able to detect changes, such as response to treatment, much more quickly (and safely) than bone scans. Several bone markers have been identified in the laboratory, but tests are not yet available for routine use.

Genetic testing

Some rare forms of breast and ovarian cancer are linked to mutations that can be detected by genetic tests. For example, 80% of women with the BRCA1, BRCA2 or TP53 mutations will develop breast cancer compared with 11% of women without these mutations. However, the most common forms of cancer are not caused by these genes, so genetic screening is only recommended for women at high risk.

Our understanding of the genetics of cancer is imperfect, so the exact meaning of genetic test results may be unclear. Counselling therefore should always be offered to help you understand and cope with the test results. Even deciding about whether or not to have the genetic tests may be hard, so you may need to talk to a specialist to help you make up your mind.

Women with the BRCA1 mutation are also at increased risk of ovarian cancer and should have annual ultrasound scans and blood tests to measure the chemical marker CA125.

Routine tests for all women

Cervical screening

This is recommended for all women aged 25–64 years who have ever had sex. Screening can detect early signs of cancer of the *cervix* (the neck of the womb), which greatly increases the chance of successful treatment. In the UK, the test, which involves taking a sample from inside the vagina, is done every 3–5 years. The cells taken from the cervix are sent to a laboratory, where they are viewed under a microscope for signs of abnormality.

Breast screening (mammography)

Viewing the breasts using a low dose X-ray (called mammography) can spot breast cancer. In the UK, all women aged 50–70 years are invited to have a mammogram every three years. This screening is also offered to older women, but there is currently no automatic invitation, so you might want to discuss this with your doctor or local breast screening unit.

Women at high risk of breast cancer because of a moderate or strong family history of breast cancer may be offered annual mammograms between the ages of 40 and 49 years (see Chapter 6). After the age of 50 years, mammograms are performed every three years – in line with the UK's National Health Service Breast Screening Programme.

The use of HRT may alter the way the breast tissue appears on a mammogram and make the breast tissue seem more dense. In most cases, this slight increase in density makes no difference, but, in theory, the denser tissue could make it harder for the doctor to see a small growth. This change in breast density may depend on the type of HRT that the woman is using. Some HRT preparations can increase the breast density seen on mammograms. Current evidence from clinical trials suggests that about one in four women who use combined HRT (oestrogen and *progestogen*) show this increase in density. Oestrogen on its own does not seem to affect the density. *Tibolone*, another form of treatment for menopausal symptoms, does not seem to have any significant effect either (for types of HRT, see Chapter 7).

It is also important to examine your own breasts for lumps and other changes. Your doctor or practice nurse can show you how to do this.

Sources of information
Journal articles

Eccles DM, Pichert G. Familial non-BRCA1/BRCA2-associated breast cancer. *Lancet Oncol* 2005; **6**: 705–11.

Fogelman I, Blake GM. Bone densitometry: an update. *Lancet* 2005; **366**: 2068–70.

Lowndes CM, Gill ON. Cervical cancer, human papillomavirus, and vaccination. *BMJ* 2005; **331**: 915–16.

Oehler MK, MacKenzie I, Kehoe S, Rees MC. Assessment of abnormal bleeding in menopausal women: an update. *J Br Menopause Soc* 2003; **9**: 117–21.

Raisz LG. Clinical practice. Screening for osteoporosis. *N Engl J Med* 2005; **353**: 164–71.

Websites

NHS Breast Screening Programme:
    www.cancerscreening.org.uk (last accessed 6 March 2006).
National Institute for Clinical Excellence (NICE):
    www.nice.org.uk (last accessed 6 March 2006).

6 Understanding your risk factors for major diseases

Cardiovascular disease
Breast cancer
Osteoporosis
Sources of information

As we age, the risk of getting certain diseases increases. Studies show that people with certain characteristics are more likely to get some diseases than others. Some of these characteristics cannot be changed – for example, your race – but others involve choices, such as what you eat and whether or not you smoke. Understanding your own risk profile can help with other decisions, such as whether or not you use hormone replacement therapy (*HRT*).

Remember that nobody can predict precisely who will get a disease. Some people with all the risk factors will stay healthy, while a few people with none of the known risk factors may develop a condition. If you are concerned about these conditions, or need more information, you should talk to your healthcare professional.

Cardiovascular disease

Because both heart attacks and strokes can be caused by narrow arteries and blood clots, some of the risk factors are similar for both (Boxes 6.1 and 6.2).

Box 6.1

Factors that increase your risk of having a heart attack (see text for details)

- Lipid (cholesterol) profile
- High blood pressure
- Smoking
- Diabetes
- Obesity
- Level of C-reactive protein
- Level of homocysteine
- Stress

Box 6.2

Factors that increase the risk of having a stroke (see text for details)

- High blood pressure (hypertension)
- Smoking
- Diabetes
- Narrowing of brain blood vessels (asymptomatic carotid stenosis)
- Atrial fibrillation
- Obesity

Risk factors for heart attacks

Lipid levels and cholesterol

High levels of fats (also called *lipids*, lipoproteins and *triglycerides*) in the blood are linked with an increased risk of heart attack for both men and women. Most people have heard of cholesterol and associate it with heart disease, but, in fact, there are several different types of cholesterol – some of which are harmful and some of which are healthy (Table 6.1).

High blood pressure (hypertension)

High blood pressure increases the risk of heart attacks in both sexes. The risk is greater in smokers and patients with diabetes, as well as those who are overweight.

Metabolic syndrome

Metabolic syndrome is a term used to describe a number of problems associated with an increased risk of heart disease. These include diabetes, high blood pressure, increased levels of lipids in blood, problems with blood clotting and obesity.

Table 6.1

Fat levels that increase the risk of heart attack

High levels	Low levels
• Low-density lipoprotein cholesterol (LDL-C) • Very low-density lipoprotein-cholesterol (VLDL-C) • Intermediate-density lipoprotein cholesterol (IDL-C) • Total cholesterol • Triglycerides • Lipoprotein a	• High-density lipoprotein cholesterol (HDL-C)

Inflammation of the blood vessels

Doctors used to believe that blocked blood vessels were entirely caused by fatty deposits, but scientists have recently shown that the walls of arteries may also get inflamed. The presence of high levels of certain chemicals in the blood, such as C-reactive protein (CRP), is linked with this type of inflammation. Women with high levels of CRP have at least five times the risk of heart problems as those with lower levels.

Homocysteine

This is a chemical marker, which is measured in the blood or from urine, that is linked with blocked arteries (*atherosclerosis*). People with homocysteine in their urine are at increased risk of vascular disease. Those who already have blocked arteries have higher levels of homocysteine in their blood.

Smoking

Smoking cigarettes is still one of the major causes of heart attacks. Smokers are between two and three times more likely to have a heart attack than non-smokers. Up to 18 in every 100 deaths from heart attacks are associated with smoking.

Depression and stress

Stress can trigger heart attacks in both sexes, while depression is linked with worse outcomes for women who have a heart attack or heart surgery.

Risk factors for stroke

High blood pressure (hypertension)

This is a major risk factor for both types of stroke (ie those caused by blood clots or by bleeding). The risk of stroke increases directly as the blood pressure rises.

Smoking

The risk of stroke in smokers is about double that in non-smokers. Eighteen in every 100 deaths from strokes are associated with smoking.

Diabetes

Having diabetes increases your risk of having a stroke by between two and six times compared with people without diabetes.

Narrowing of the carotid arteries (carotid stenosis)

The carotid arteries carry blood to the brain. Narrowing of these arteries is termed carotid stenosis. Unlike narrowing of the *coronary* arteries, which may cause pain (angina) or other symptoms, many people with carotid stenosis are unaware of the problem, as it does not cause any symptoms. The carotid arteries in about one in 16 women (5–7%) and up to one in 10 men older than 65 years are less than half their normal size. This increases the risk of stroke.

Heart rhythm problems

Problems with the heart beat are termed arrhythmia. One common type of *arrhythmia* involves problems with the main heart chambers or atria and is termed atrial fibrillation. This condition is thought to cause about half of all strokes caused by blood clots. About one in 20 people with atrial fibrillation will have a stroke over the course of a single year.

High lipid levels (hyperlipidaemia)

The link between raised lipid levels (eg cholesterol) in the blood and the risk of stroke is less direct and clear than the link with heart attacks. Some large studies have found no link between levels of cholesterol and the rate of stroke. However, medicines called *statins*, which are used to lower lipid levels, reduce the risk of both heart attacks and strokes.

Obesity

Being seriously overweight (obese) increases your risk of both heart attacks and strokes.

Breast cancer

Factors that increase the risk of getting breast cancer include (Table 6.2):

- not having children (compared with women who have children)
- having your first child later in life (compared with having a baby earlier)

Table 6.2

Increased risk of breast cancer with different risk factors

Risk factor	Increase in breast cancer risk
Periods starting before age 11 years	1.50 times increase
Menopause after age 55 years	2.00 times increase
Postmenopausal obesity	1.60 times increase
Not having a child before age 30 years	1.90 times increase
Alcohol (more than 2–3 units per day)	1.50 times increase
HRT containing oestrogen and progesterone for more than five years	1.24 times increase (see Chapter 8)
HRT containing oestrogen alone for more than five years	1–1.24 times increase (see Chapter 8)

- being overweight
- having a family history of breast cancer.

Family history of breast cancer

To get information about diseases that run in families, doctors may ask about your relatives. Remember that the doctor only wants to know about your blood relatives – **not** those who have married into your family (such as your sister-in-law or your uncle's wife). Family links are sometimes referred to as 'first degree', 'second degree' and 'third degree':

- first-degree relatives: mother, father, daughter, son, sister or brother
- second-degree relatives: grandparents, grandchildren, aunt, uncle, niece, nephew, half-brother or half-sister
- third-degree relatives: great grandparents, great grandchildren, great aunt, great uncle, first cousin, grand nephew and grand niece.

Box 6.3

Clinical guidance for the classification and care of women at risk of familial breast cancer. Adapted from NICE (2004) Familial breast cancer. Quick reference guide

Women likely to be at moderate risk (ie lifetime risk between 17% and less than 30%)
- One 1st degree relative diagnosed before age 40 years
- One 1st degree relative and one 2nd degree relative diagnosed after average age 50 years
- Two 1st degree relatives diagnosed after average age 50 years

Women likely to be at more than moderate risk (ie lifetime risk of more than 30%)
Female breast cancer only
- One 1st degree relative and one 2nd degree relative diagnosed before average age 50 years
- Two 1st degree relatives diagnosed before average age of 50 years
- Three or more 1st or 2nd degree relatives diagnosed at any age

Male breast cancer
- One 1st degree male relative diagnosed at any age

Bilateral breast cancer (cancer in both breasts)
- One 1st degree relative where the first primary cancer diagnosed before age 50 years

Breast and ovarian cancer
- One 1st or 2nd degree relative with ovarian cancer at any age **and** one 1st or 2nd degree relative with breast cancer at any age (one should be a 1st degree relative)

If your doctor considers you to be at moderate or greater risk than the average woman as a result of your family history, they would consider referring you to a specialist.

Being at risk of breast cancer means that there is a possibility that the person will develop the disease, but it does not mean it will necessarily happen. Women are regarded as at or near population risk if their risk of developing breast cancer between the ages of 40 and 50 years is estimated at less than 3% (three women in 100) and their lifetime risk is estimated at less than 17% (17 women in 100) (Box 6.3).

Osteoporosis

Factors that increase the risk of *osteoporosis* (brittle bones) are shown in Table 6.3. These can be used as a guide for the need to measure your bone mineral density (see Chapter 5).

Table 6.3

Factors that increase the risk of osteoporosis (brittle bones)

Type of factor	Example
Genetic	Family history of fracture, particularly hip fracture (especially mother or sister)
Constitutional	Low body weight
	Early menopause (younger than 45 years)
Lifestyle	Cigarette smoking
	Alcohol abuse
	Low calcium intake
	Sedentary lifestyle (not enough exercise)
Medicines	Glucocorticosteroids (>5 mg prednisolone or equivalent per day)
Diseases	Rheumatoid arthritis
	Neuromuscular disease
	Chronic liver disease
	Malabsorption syndromes
	Hyperparathyroidism (overactive parathyroid)
	Hyperthyroidism (overactive thyroid)
	Hypogonadism (underdeveloped reproductive organs)

Sources of information

Journal articles

Huxley R, Barzi F, Woodward M. Excess risk of fatal coronary heart disease associated with diabetes in men and women: meta-analysis of 37 prospective cohort studies. *BMJ* 2006; **332**: 73–8.

Kaplan NM, Opie LH. Controversies in hypertension. *Lancet* 2006; **367**: 168–76.

Siris ES, Brenneman SK, Barrett-Connor E *et al.* The effect of age and bone mineral density on the absolute, excess, and relative risk of fracture in postmenopausal women aged 50–99: results from the National Osteoporosis Risk Assessment (NORA). *Osteoporos Int* 2006; **17**: 565–74.

Websites

American Cancer Society:
www.cancer.org (last accessed 6 March 2006).
British Heart Foundation·
www.bhf.org.uk (last accessed 6 March 2006).
National Institute for Clinical Excellence (NICE):
www.nice.org.uk (last accessed 6 March 2006).

7 Hormone replacement therapy

Over 50 forms of hormone replacement therapy (*HRT*) are currently available in the UK. They offer different doses, combinations and routes of taking the hormones.

What is HRT?

Most problems of the menopause are the result of the sudden fall in levels of the female sex hormone *oestrogen*. The fundamental idea of HRT therefore is to replace the lost oestrogen. However, giving oestrogen alone can harm the womb lining (*endometrium*) in women who have not had a *hysterectomy*. So, women who have not had a hysterectomy need a second hormone, called a *progestogen*, to balance the effects of oestrogen on the endometrium. Hormone replacement therapy can be delivered *orally* (tablets), *transdermally* (through the skin), subcutaneously (a long-lasting implant), intranasally (sniffed) or vaginally.

Oestrogens

Note: this book uses British spellings, but you may see the American spelling 'estrogen' in other places, such as websites. If you are searching for information about HRT on the Internet, try using both spellings.

Oestrogens are sometimes classified as 'natural' or 'synthetic', but these terms can be confusing. In this book, we use the term 'natural' oestrogens to refer to compounds that can be found naturally in the body – even when they have been manufactured in a laboratory of a pharmaceutical company. These include oestradiol, oestrone and oestriol, which are usually prepared from extracts of soya beans or yams. Horse (equine) urine is another common source of HRT hormones; equine oestrogens include about 50–65% oestrone sulphate (the same as the human form), but the remainder are animal oestrogens, such as equilin sulphate (which does not occur naturally in humans). Synthetic oestrogens, such as *ethinyl oestradiol* and mestranol, which are used in contraceptive pills, are less suitable for HRT than natural oestrogens, because they have a more powerful effect on the body's metabolism.

Table 7.1 shows the lowest doses that are generally thought to offer protection from *osteoporosis*, although increasing evidence suggests that lower doses may be just as effective and may cause fewer side-effects. However, young women who have an induced (surgical) menopause at first may require higher doses to control menopausal symptoms.

Table 7.1
Minimum bone-sparing doses of HRT

Oestrogen	Preparation	Minimum dose (per day except for implants)
Oestradiol	Oral	1–2 mg
Oestradiol	Patch	25–50 µg
Oestradiol	Gel	1–5 g depending on preparation
Oestradiol	Implant	50 mg (every six months)
Conjugated equine oestrogens	Oral	0.3–0.6 mg

Progestogens

Progestogens are chemicals that share many properties with the female hormone *progesterone*, which is produced by the ovaries (see Chapter 1). Most progestogens are made from plant sources such as yams. There are two main groups of progestogens: those similar to progesterone (*dydrogesterone* and *medroxyprogesterone acetate*) and those based on *testosterone* (norethisterone and *levonorgestrel*). A new progestogen called *drospirenone* is now used in

HRT. Progestogens are currently given mainly as tablets, but norethisterone and levonorgestrel are available in transdermal patches combined with oestradiol, and levonorgestrel can be delivered directly to the womb via an intrauterine device (IUD) (see Chapter 4). The naturally occurring type of progesterone is available as a vaginal gel but availability varies worldwide. A progesterone pessary for vaginal or rectal use is produced but is not currently licensed for HRT.

Tibolone

Tibolone is a synthetic steroid that has similar effects to both the female hormones oestrogen and progestogen and also the male hormones, which are known as *androgens*. It is a 'no bleed' form of HRT. It can improve psychological and *vasomotor* symptoms (hot flushes and night sweats) and can increase sex drive (*libido*). It can also prevent osteoporosis; the bone-sparing dose is 2.5 mg per day. It is a good form of HRT for postmenopausal women who do not want to continue to have periods.

Androgens (male hormones)

The male hormone testosterone may be prescribed to improve a woman's sex drive (libido). However, this treatment is not always successful because sexual problems around the menopause are often caused by several different factors. The current form of treatment is an implant, but testosterone patches and gels are being studied in research trials.

HRT after a hysterectomy

One in five British women will have had a hysterectomy by the time they are aged 52 years. The best HRT for women who have had a total hysterectomy, in which the whole womb including its neck (*cervix*) has been removed, is oestrogen alone. Combined HRT (oestrogen plus progestogen) offers no benefits for these women and may increase their risk of breast cancer. However, women who have had a partial (subtotal) hysterectomy may still have some womb lining (endometrium) present. This will respond to oestrogen alone (see below). To decide whether or not this is the case, they may be given sequential HRT first. If they have monthly bleeds, this is an indication that there is some womb lining present. In this case, they should receive combined HRT.

HRT for women who have not had a hysterectomy

Women who have not had a hysterectomy need both oestrogen and progestogen. The progestogen is added to reduce the risk of benign but excessive growth (*endometrial hyperplasia*) and cancer of the womb lining (endometrium), which can be caused by oestrogen alone. Progestogen may be taken cyclically (for 10 to 14 days every month or every three months) or continuously (Table 7.2).

Women who have had endometrial ablation (an operation to destroy the endometrium that is often performed in women who have heavy periods) should receive progestogen. This is because not all of the endometrium will necessarily have been removed, so they may be at risk of hyperplasia or cancer if they take oestrogen alone.

Table 7.2

Effect on bleeding of the timing of progestogen in HRT

Timing of progestogen	Effect on bleeding
10–14 days every four weeks	Monthly bleeds
14 days every 13 weeks	Bleeds every three months
Continuous (every day)	No bleeds

HRT around the menopause

Women often notice hot flushes, mood changes and vaginal dryness several months or years before their periods stop (see Chapter 2). You do not need to wait for your periods to stop before starting HRT. The best options at this stage are usually monthly cyclic treatments with oestrogen every day plus progestogen for 10–14 days each month. Women with infrequent periods and those who get side-effects from progestogens may prefer to take the progestogen every three months; this is called long-cycle HRT. Continuous combined HRT preparations that give both oestrogen and progestogen every day are not recommended around the menopause, because they are likely to cause irregular bleeding.

HRT after the menopause

One year after the menopause has occurred, many women prefer to switch to continuous combined HRT, as this does not cause any bleeding and may reduce the risk of endometrial cancer. This form of HRT is sometimes called 'no bleed' HRT. However, it is not always easy for doctors to decide when a woman has reached this stage. Strictly speaking, a woman is considered to be postmenopausal 12 months after her last period, but this can be difficult to determine, especially for women who start to use HRT before their periods stop.

Irregular bleeding or spotting can occur during the first 4–6 months of continuous combined HRT and is not a cause for alarm. However, you should consult your doctor if you get heavy (rather than light) bleeding, if bleeding lasts for more than six months or if bleeding starts suddenly after some time without bleeding. Irregular bleeding may sometimes be improved by increasing the amount of progestogen.

HRT delivery systems that raise hormone levels throughout the body (systemic HRT)

Any medicine taken by mouth (orally) will go into the stomach and intestines, be absorbed and pass into the liver. This process causes chemical changes to the medicine before it reaches the bloodstream. If a medicine is delivered directly into the bloodstream (*parenterally*), these changes are avoided. The route of delivery therefore can influence the effects of medicines and also their side-effects. Parenteral delivery systems include skin patches and gels, nasal sprays, vaginal rings and implants. Both oral and parenteral systems raise hormone levels throughout the body (Box 7.1).

Box 7.1

HRT delivery systems

- Orally as tablets
- Transdermally (through the skin): patches and gels
- Implants beneath the skin
- Nasal sprays
- Vaginal rings
- Intrauterine devices

Oral versus parenteral systems

When HRT is taken orally as tablets, the main type of oestrogen in the bloodstream is oestrone. When HRT is taken parenterally, the main hormone is oestradiol. Other differences between oral and parenteral HRT are complex and subtle, and their effects are controversial. Laboratory tests suggest that the route of delivery might affect blood clotting and levels of *lipids* (ie cholesterol), but the actual effect on women taking different types of HRT is unclear.

Doctors currently debate the advantages of oral and parenteral administration of HRT. There is no clear evidence that one route is better than the other. Many doctors recommend tablets as the first choice for most women, unless there is a special reason to prefer another form. However, some will recommend parenteral preparations.

Transdermal systems: patches and gels

Oestradiol and progestogens can pass into the bloodstream through the skin (transdermally). They can therefore be delivered via transdermal patches or gels. There are two types of HRT patch. Reservoir patches contain hormone in an alcohol-based solution and stick to the skin by an adhesive ring at the edge of the patch. Matrix patches contain hormone distributed throughout an adhesive layer that covers the whole of the patch. Allergic skin reactions are less common with matrix patches than with reservoir patches.

Implants

Small pellets of oestradiol can be placed just under the skin. The insertion is carried out under local anaesthetic. These implants release oestradiol over many months. Implants have the advantage that you do not have to remember to take medication. However, some women find that their menopausal symptoms return even though the implant is still releasing oestradiol. Others do not like the idea of an implant that may have an effect for many years. Levels of oestradiol in the blood may be checked before new pellets are inserted, especially in women who go back more frequently for treatment.

Nasal sprays

Oestradiol can be given by a nasal spray and is quickly absorbed into the bloodstream (in 10–30 minutes). A daily intranasal dose of 300 μg oestradiol seems to be as good as taking 2 mg/day tablets for treating menopausal symptoms.

Vaginal rings

Because oestradiol is so well absorbed, some vaginal rings can give blood levels similar to tablets or patches.

Intrauterine devices

Devices placed in the *uterus* (IUDs, sometimes called coils) may be used before the menopause as contraceptives. One type of IUD releases the progestogen levonorgestrel (see Chapter 4). As well as being a contraceptive, it can therefore be used to deliver progestogen for HRT. The contraceptive effects may be useful in the perimenopause, when women are often still fertile despite having menopausal symptoms. Another advantage is that this method of delivering progestogen is the only method that may not cause bleeding in perimenopausal women.

Managing the side-effects of HRT

Although HRT aims to replace naturally occurring hormones, it can cause side-effects. Women who start HRT when their natural oestrogen levels have become very low may get side-effects simply because their bodies have got used to these low hormone levels. Many of these effects will wear off as the body becomes used to the treatment.

The oestrogen in HRT can cause bloating (fluid retention), tender or swollen breasts, nausea, headaches, leg cramps and indigestion. Progestogen may also cause fluid retention, tender breasts and headache. Some women also report migraines, mood swings, depression, acne, lower abdominal pain (belly ache) and backache.

If you think your HRT is causing a side-effect, you should discuss this with your doctor. Some side-effects wear off over time, such as breast tenderness, while others may be helped by taking a lower dose, a different type of HRT or a different formulation (for example, patches instead of tablets).

Many women put on weight around the menopause and, if they are using HRT, sometimes think this is to blame. However, scientific studies have found no evidence that HRT causes weight gain.

Bleeding

If you take sequential or cyclical HRT, you will normally get a predictable pattern of light bleeding towards the end or soon after the end of the progestogen phase. Tell your doctor if you have bleeding that is heavy, longer than usual, irregular or painful. Changing the type or dose of progestogen may help this, but your doctor will also need to check that there is no other cause. A few women who use sequential HRT (about 5%) have no bleeding, and it is not a reason to worry. No bleeding is usually due to the womb lining being very thin, but if you are in the perimenopause, you should also make sure that you are not pregnant (see the section on contraception in Chapter 4).

Breakthrough bleeding (bleeding at unexpected times) is common with both continuous combined and long-cycle (three-monthly progestogen) HRT in the first 3–6 months of treatment. Tell your doctor if you get breakthrough bleeding after this time.

How long should you take HRT?

If the main reason for taking HRT is hot flushes and night sweats, you will probably need to take it for about five years. Taking HRT for this length of time does not seriously increase your risk of breast cancer. After about five years, your doctor may suggest you stop the HRT to see if the symptoms come back. Although hot flushes usually stop after 2–5 years, some women will experience symptoms for many years – even into their 70s and 80s.

If the main reason for taking HRT is to preserve bone strength (and prevent osteoporosis), however, you should consider taking HRT for life, because bones start to weaken as soon as you stop treatment. Studies suggest that taking HRT for only 5–10 years around the menopause (when most women are in their 50s) does not protect against breaking your hip when you are aged 80 years.

How long you take HRT is a personal choice, and you should discuss this with your doctor. Some women are happy to take HRT for life, while others might want to switch to other treatments that can help with brittle bones, such as a bisphosphonate (see Chapter 9). Doctors now think that taking combined HRT (ie oestrogen plus progestogen) for a long time slightly increases the risk of developing breast cancer. Deciding how long to take HRT may therefore depend on your feelings about this risk and whether or not you have other risk factors for breast cancer (see Chapter 6).

Women who have an early (premature) menopause are usually advised to take HRT until the normal age for menopause (ie until they are aged 52 years). After this, the choice about whether or not to take HRT will depend on the same factors as for other women, as discussed above.

How to stop HRT

No clear evidence shows whether or not it is better to stop HRT gradually. Menopausal symptoms such as hot flushes sometimes return when HRT is stopped suddenly. Older women seem to need lower doses of HRT to control symptoms than younger women, so it might be logical to switch to a lower dose before stopping. This is something to discuss with your doctor.

Treating local symptoms without raising hormone levels throughout the body

Some women do not wish to use, or cannot take, *systemic* HRT (any form that raises hormone levels throughout the body), but they still appreciate relief of symptoms, such as dry vagina and urinary problems. In this case, oestrogens can be given locally to the vagina in the form of a low-dose cream, pessary, tablet or ring. These preparations raise local hormone levels but do not affect the whole body. Low doses of natural (rather than synthetic) oestrogens (eg oestriol or oestradiol) are best for this form of treatment. Progestogen is not needed, as these local doses of oestrogen do not affect the endometrium. Synthetic oestrogens should be avoided, because they can enter the bloodstream from the vagina. Long-term treatment is usually needed, as symptoms often return when treatment is stopped.

Sources of information

Journal articles

Grady D, Sawaya GF. Discontinuation of postmenopausal hormone therapy. *Am J Med* 2005; **118** (12 Suppl 2): 163–5.

Liu JH. Therapeutic effects of progestins, androgens, and tibolone for menopausal symptoms. *Am J Med* 2005; **118** (12 Suppl 2): 88–92.

Nelson HD. Commonly used types of postmenopausal estrogen for treatment of hot flashes: scientific review. *JAMA* 2004; **291**: 1610–20.

Ockene JK, Barad DH, Cochrane BB *et al.* Symptom experience after discontinuing use of estrogen plus progestin. *JAMA* 2005; **294**: 183–93.

Suckling J, Lethaby A, Kennedy R. Local oestrogen for vaginal atrophy in postmenopausal women. *Cochrane Database Syst Rev* 2003; **(4)**: CD001500.

Books

Monthly Index of Medical Specialties. London: Haymarket Medical, 2006 (published monthly).

British Medical Association, Royal Pharmaceutical Society of Great Britain. *British National Formulary*. London: BMA, RPS, 2006.

Websites

British National Formulary (updated twice yearly):
www.bnf.org/bnf/ (last accessed 6 March 2006).
PRODIGY Knowledge:
www.prodigy.nhs.uk (last accessed 6 March 2006).

8 Hormone replacement therapy: benefits, risks and controversies

Understanding the evidence
Types of clinical trials
What does 'risk' mean?
Recent major clinical trials of HRT
Benefits of HRT
Risks of HRT
Uncertainties about HRT
Tibolone
Sources of information

Understanding the evidence

Information about the benefits and risks of using hormone replacement therapy (*HRT*) comes from clinical studies. In order to understand what the results of these studies really mean, you need to understand something about the studies themselves. In particular, the results of two large studies have caused controversy about HRT among health professionals and women and have been widely reported in the media. These studies are the Women's Health Initiative (WHI) and the Million Women Study (MWS). This chapter aims to help you understand them.

Types of clinical trials

Primary and secondary prevention trials

Hormone replacement therapy may be taken to prevent a condition such as *osteoporosis* developing in women who are currently healthy; this is called primary prevention. Another reason for taking HRT is to reduce the dangers of an existing condition – for example, to reduce the risk of fracture in women who already have osteoporosis; this is called secondary prevention. It is important to know whether or not a trial studied healthy women or those who already had a disease, as their responses to treatment might vary.

Randomized, cohort and case–control studies

Many early studies of HRT simply compared the health of women who used HRT with those who did not. The problem with this method is that you do not know whether or not differences between the groups are really caused by HRT or whether or not other factors are important. For example, women who use HRT might be more health conscious and therefore have a better diet and take more exercise than those who do not use HRT.

Randomized trials are an attempt to avoid this problem, which is sometimes called the 'healthy user bias'. A randomized trial studies a group of patients who are randomly allocated to receive HRT or another treatment. If you look at enough patients, it should not matter whether or not some are healthier than others because each group will contain a mixture of the different types of patient. However, even very large randomized trials are not perfect, because you never know about the patients who chose not to enter the study. When a doctor and patient are choosing the best treatment, they have to decide whether or not the results of a study can be expected to apply to the individual's own situation. For example, the WHI study looked at women older than 50 years, but we do not know whether or not the results apply to women with an earlier menopause.

In addition, randomized trials tend to be short term, and some treatments may take several years to have an effect. Another problem is that patients in a trial may behave differently from normal – for example, they might take their medicines more conscientiously. Some of these problems can be overcome by cohort studies.

Cohort studies can be thought of as natural experiments. They can study large groups of diverse people over long periods and provide information about a number of outcomes, including rare side-effects. Cohort studies are similar to randomized trials, in that they compare outcomes in groups that did and did not receive a treatment. The main difference is that the decision about whether or not one person gets the treatment does not depend on chance. Therefore, differences between the two groups may not be the result of the treatment but the result of other factors.

To overcome the problem of differences in risk factors between groups, a **case–control design** may be used. In a case–control study, patients with a particular disease (called cases) are identified and 'matched' with people who do not have the disease, but are similar to them in other ways (called controls). For example, if you think smoking might affect the outcome you are studying, you would compare non-smoking cases with non-smoking controls.

Cohort studies and case–control studies are examples of observational study designs. The problem with all observational studies is that they may show relationships between a factor and an illness or outcome, but they cannot prove that this was the cause.

What does 'risk' mean?

Studies often report their results as **relative risks**; however, this can be hard to understand. For example, a relative risk of 2 could describe something that increases the risk of a disease from one in a million to two in a million or something that increases the risk of a disease from four people in 10 to eight people in 10. In order to understand what a relative risk means, you therefore have to know how common a disease is (which is known as the **absolute risk**).

Relative risks only describe the size of the increase in risk without telling you how large the absolute risk is. Thus, a small increase in relative risk for a common disease (large absolute risk) can have a big effect on the number of people affected, but a larger increase in relative risk for a very rare event (small absolute risk) will have only a tiny impact on the number affected.

Ways of expressing risk

Risks of treatments can be expressed as a ratio that compares the risk in those who took the treatment with the risk in those who did not. In particular, you may see the terms **hazard ratio** (or HR) and **odds ratio** (or OR). An HR of 0.5 is the same as saying the relative risk of something happening in one group is half that in the other group. In order to understand an HR, you therefore need to know the absolute risk. The OR is the chance of something happening in the treated group expressed as a proportion of the odds of that event happening in the untreated group.

Recent major clinical trials of HRT

The two major trials that have caused controversy among the medical profession are the Women's Health Initiative (WHI) and the Million Women Study (MWS). They do not agree on the risk of HRT containing *oestrogen* alone on breast cancer (see below). This disagreement may be because of the different designs of these studies.

Women's Health Initiative (WHI)

The WHI is a large and complex series of studies focusing on the major health problems faced by postmenopausal women, including cancer, heart disease and osteoporosis. It studies not only the effect of HRT but also lifestyle factors such as low fat diets and calcium and vitamin D supplements. It involves American women aged between 50 and 79 years with an average age of about 62. It includes randomized and observational studies.

Million Women Study (MWS)

The MWS was an observational study of the effects of different types of HRT on the risk of breast cancer. It was run in the UK and used information from women attending the National Health Service Breast Screening Programme, who completed a questionnaire. As the name suggests, the MWS studied just more than one million women – about half of whom had used HRT at some time. Some of the findings of the MWS are unexpected, and this has led some experts to question the way the study was performed. For example:

- The study reported lower risks of breast cancer in postmenopausal women than premenopausal women, despite the well-established fact that the risk of breast cancer increases with age.
- The study only asked women about their use of HRT at the start of the study and did not record whether or not they changed preparations or stopped HRT during the study follow-up period.
- Many women who had not had a *hysterectomy* reported using an HRT containing only oestrogen (which should only be prescribed for those who have had a hysterectomy).

Box 8.1

Benefits, risks and uncertainties of HRT

Benefits
Relief of hot flushes
Relief from vaginal dryness, urinary frequency/urgency and recurrent urinary tract infections
Improvement of sex drive (libido) or other sexual problems (sometimes in combination with testosterone)
Reduced risk of fractures associated with osteoporosis (brittle bones), particularly spine and hip fractures
Reduced risk of bowel (colorectal) cancer

Risks
Breast cancer
Endometrial cancer (womb lining)
Deep blood clots (venous thromboembolism)
Gallbladder problems

Uncertainties
Cardiovascular disease (heart disease and stroke)
Dementia
Alzheimer's disease
Ovarian cancer

Box 8.1 lists the benefits, risk and uncertainties shown by these studies, which are described in detail in the text below.

Benefits of HRT

Vasomotor symptoms

Relief of *vasomotor* symptoms (eg hot flushes) is the most common reason for prescribing HRT. Good evidence from randomized studies, including WHI, shows that oestrogen can treat hot flushes. Improvement is usually noted in four weeks.

The maximum effect of any type of HRT is usually seen by three months, so this is a good point to review the treatment. The HRT should be continued for at least one year, otherwise symptoms often recur.

Changes in urinary and reproductive organs (urogenital atrophy)

The changes that take place in the urinary and reproductive tissues after the menopause are called urogenital *atrophy*. They can cause symptoms such as vaginal dryness, urinary frequency and urgency, and recurrent urinary tract infections (see Chapter 3). These symptoms respond well to oestrogens, but improvement may take several months.

However, incontinence (eg leaking urine when you exercise, laugh, cough or sneeze) does not respond to *systemic* HRT. Loss of sex drive (*libido*) and other sexual problems may be improved by oestrogen, but they may also need *testosterone*, especially in younger women who have had their ovaries removed. At present, testosterone is available only as an implant for use in women; patches and gels are in development.

Osteoporosis (brittle bones)

Evidence from randomized controlled trials (including WHI) shows that HRT reduces the risk of spine and hip fractures, as well as other fractures caused by osteoporosis. However, as with any decision about treatment, you and your doctor must weigh up the risks and benefits of long-term use. Other treatments for osteoporosis (such as *bisphosphonates*) may be more suitable than HRT, especially for older women, but there is not much information about their use in younger (eg perimenopausal) women (see Chapter 9).

Some women have no bone response despite taking HRT as recommended, but the reasons for this are uncertain. Women who smoke or are very thin seem to be most likely not to respond.

Bowel (colorectal) cancer

Some studies have suggested that HRT reduces the risk of bowel cancer by about one-third. This effect was also seen among women who took combined oestrogen–progestogen HRT in the WHI study but not among those who took oestrogen-only HRT. There is no information about the effects of HRT in high-risk populations, and little is known about the risk of *colorectal cancer* when treatment is stopped.

Risks of HRT

As we have seen, HRT offers many benefits. Yet, as with any medicine, it also carries risks. When deciding whether or not to use HRT, you need to weigh up the benefits and the risks and think about how they apply to you individually.

The three major risks linked with HRT are:

* breast cancer
* endometrial cancer, which affects the lining of the womb
* deep venous blood clots (venous thromboembolic disease).

Risk of developing breast cancer

Breast cancer is a common disease, with a lifetime risk in the United Kingdom of one in nine. It is currently the most common cancer to affect women. Most breast cancers (80%) are found in women older than 50 years. Understandably, women are concerned about any factors that may increase their risk, and this is the most common reason given for not wanting to use HRT for long periods. However, the proportion of women who survive breast cancer has increased considerably over the past 20 years. This is mainly the result of the more widespread use of effective therapies and the introduction of mammographic screening. This means that most women diagnosed with breast cancer will be alive five years after diagnosis. The estimated relative five-year survival rate for women diagnosed in England and Wales in 2001–03 was 80% but only 52% for women diagnosed in 1971–5. The estimated relative 20-year survival rate for women with breast cancer has increased from 44% in the early 1990s to 64% for the most recent period (Figure 8.1).

The risk of developing breast cancer increases with age, but the pattern is interesting. Before the menopause, the rate increases steeply, but after the menopause, the increase is less rapid. This suggests that sex hormones have a role. Women who naturally have a late menopause are therefore at greater risk of breast cancer than those who have an earlier menopause. The use of HRT seems to carry a similar risk as having a late natural menopause. The risk also decreases when HRT is stopped, and five years after stopping HRT, the risk of breast cancer is the same as for women who have never used HRT.

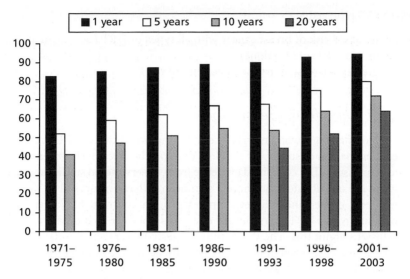

Figure 8.1 Age-standardized relative survival for patients diagnosed with breast cancer, England and Wales, 1971–2003. Adapted with permission from Cancer Research UK, http://info.cancerresearchuk. org/cancerstats/types/breast/survival/?a=5441 (last accessed 6 March 2006)

The risk of breast cancer seems to depend on the type of HRT. This had been found in several studies published before the WHI and MWS studies. Overall, combined HRT containing oestrogen and progestogen seems to carry a slightly higher risk than oestrogen alone, but this must be balanced against the other risks of unopposed oestrogen in women who have not had a hysterectomy.

The effect of other factors known to increase the risk of breast cancer – such as not having children, having your first baby late in life, being overweight and having close relatives with breast cancer – may be greater than the increased risk observed with HRT.

The WHI study found:

- Women who took HRT in the form of equine oestrogen (with no added progestogen) were 23% less likely to develop breast cancer than those who took no HRT (but received a dummy tablet or *placebo*). This worked out at about five fewer cases of breast cancer per 1000 women aged 50–70 years.
- An increased risk of developing breast cancer was only seen in women who used combined HRT for at least three years and who had used HRT before the study. This worked out at about four extra cases per 1000 women aged 50–70 years.

The MWS reported:

- an increased risk of breast cancer with all types of HRT (oestrogen alone, combined HRT and tibolone)
- the greatest increase in risk with combined HRT.

Risk of dying from breast cancer

As well as affecting a woman's risk of developing breast cancer, HRT may also affect her chances of survival if she does develop the disease. However, this is hard to measure. The combined evidence from observational studies suggests that the use of HRT does not have a significant effect on survival in women with breast cancer and may even increase it. In contrast, MWS reported poorer survival in HRT users, but the effect was not clear, so it is hard to draw conclusions about this. The WHI study suggested a very small unfavourable (1.5%) effect on survival difference at 10 years between combined HRT users and non-users. This equates to an extra 1.4 deaths per 1000 women with a history of using combined HRT at the time of diagnosis. The theoretical risk of taking oestrogen alone will be lower.

Endometrial cancer

Endometrial cancer is much rarer than breast cancer, with fewer than one in 1000 women in the UK older than 50 years developing this disease. The link between unopposed oestrogen replacement therapy and endometrial cancer was established more than 20 years ago. Use of unopposed oestrogen for 10 years increases the risk of endometrial cancer almost 10 times, and the increased risk remains after the oestrogen is stopped. Women who have not had a hysterectomy therefore are usually prescribed a combined preparation of oestrogen and progestogen. This has been shown to reduce the risk of both benign and cancerous growths of the womb lining (*endometrium*). Continuous combined preparations (oestrogen and progestogen both taken all the time) do not seem to cause any increase in the risk of endometrial cancer, but there may still be a slight increase if the progestogen is not taken all the time.

Women with diabetes and women who are obese have an increased risk of endometrial cancer. This increase is larger than that seen with HRT.

The main symptoms of endometrial cancer are heavy or unexpected bleeding. You should therefore tell your doctor if you experience these while using any form of HRT. You should also tell your doctor if you have any unexpected bleeding after the menopause – even if you are not taking HRT.

Deep blood clots (venous thromboembolism)

Venous thromboembolism (or VTE) occurs when veins become blocked by blood clots. Although we have known for some time that the contraceptive pill increases the risk of VTE, a link with HRT was shown only in 1996. The baseline risk of VTE in women older than 50 years who are not using HRT is just under two per 1000. For every 100 women who develop VTE, one or two will die. The use of HRT increases the risk of getting a VTE between two and three times. This increase is slightly less than that for many oral contraceptives. There is some evidence that *transdermal* HRT (patches or gels) carry less risk than tablets. The highest risk occurs in the first year of use.

Other factors that increase the risk of developing VTE are advancing age, obesity and blood clotting diseases such as Factor V Leiden thrombophilia. Women who have previously had a VTE have an increased risk of developing another during the first year of HRT use.

Gallbladder problems

Two large studies – WHI and HERS (the Heart and Estrogen/progestin Replacement Study) – have reported higher rates of gallbladder disease among women using HRT. In developed countries, at least 20% of women over 60 have gallstones but never have a problem. Gallbladder problems are also known to increase with age and obesity.

Uncertainties about HRT

Cardiovascular disease (CVD)

Heart attacks and strokes are a major cause of death in women. It is therefore important to know the effects of HRT on these two diseases. Until the late 1990s, most doctors believed that oestrogen reduced the risk of heart disease. Cohort studies suggested that HRT reduced the risk of *coronary* heart disease by 40–50%. There seemed to be no difference between the use of oestrogen alone and oestrogen combined with progestogen.

There were concerns that the apparent benefits of HRT were because of healthy women taking part in the studies. However, research showed that it did have benefits for postmenopausal women with existing heart disease. The greatest benefits in terms of survival were seen in women with the most severe coronary *artery* disease. However, these beneficial results have not been confirmed by randomized controlled trials such as WHI and HERS, but this may have been due to the dose and type of HRT used. The timing of HRT may also be critical in determining *cardiovascular* effects, as found in the WHI and prospective large observational cohort Nurses' Health Study for both oestrogen alone and combined HRT. For example women in the WHI who started combined HRT within 10 years of the menopause had a lower risk of *CHD* than women who started later (more than 20 years after the menopause) (Figure 8.2).

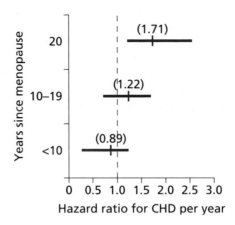

Figure 8.2 Influence of time since menopause on effect of combined hormone replacement therapy on coronary heart disease (CHD). Adapted from Manson *et al.* (2003)

A large observational study (the Nurses' Health Study) showed no increase in the rate of stroke with HRT, except in women taking high-dose oestrogen. The randomized HERS trial reported no increase in stroke for women using HRT. However, women taking HRT in the WHI study had more *ischaemic strokes* (those due to blood clots) but no more *haemorrhagic strokes* (the type due to bleeding) than women who took placebo (Table 8.1).

Several randomized trials have shown that HRT does not improve survival or prevent another stroke in women who have already had an ischaemic stroke.

Table 8.1

Increased risk of stroke expressed as extra cases per 10,000 women per year compared with women who did not receive HRT in the WHI study

Age (years)	Combined HRT	Oestrogen-only HRT
50–59	4	0
60–69	9	19
70–79	13	14

Dementia and Alzheimer's disease

One in 10 retired people will develop *dementia* (or a serious loss of mental function), and this rises to one in five people older than 80 years. Alzheimer's disease is more common in women than men, and women also live longer. Observational studies and animal experiments have suggested that oestrogen may delay or reduce the risk of developing Alzheimer's disease, but HRT does not seem to improve established disease. However, women who received HRT in the WHI study were twice as likely to develop dementia as those who did not receive hormones. This finding was surprising, and the cause is not known. We therefore need more evidence before we can draw firm conclusions about the effects of HRT on dementia.

Ovarian cancer

Use of combined HRT (oestrogen and progestogen) does not seem to increase the risk of cancer of the ovaries. However, there may be an increased risk linked to very long-term use of oestrogen alone, but the effects have only been seen in women who took oestrogen for at least 10 years.

Tibolone

Tibolone is often classed as a type of HRT. It is effective in treating menopausal symptoms such as hot flushes. Although it helps maintain bone density, we do not know yet whether or not it prevents fractures. It shares some of the risks of oestrogen-based HRT, and the MWS showed an increased risk of breast and endometrial cancer. There is not enough information to say whether or not tibolone affects the risk of VTE in the same way as other types of HRT.

However, information from randomized trials is awaited.

Sources of information

Journal articles

Barnabei VM, Cochrane BB, Aragaki AK *et al.* Menopausal symptoms and treatment-related effects of estrogen and progestin in the Women's Health Initiative. *Obstet Gynecol* 2005; **105**: 1063–73.

Beral V, Bull D, Reeves G. Endometrial cancer and hormone-replacement therapy in the Million Women Study. *Lancet* 2005; **365**: 1543–51.

Gabriel SR, Carmona L, Roque M *et al.* Hormone replacement therapy for preventing cardiovascular disease in post-menopausal women. *Cochrane Database Syst Rev* 2005; **(2)**: CD002229.

Grady D, Herrington D, Bittner V *et al*; HERS Research Group. Cardiovascular disease outcomes during 6.8 years of hormone therapy: Heart and Estrogen/progestin Replacement Study follow-up (HERS II). *JAMA* 2002; **288**: 49–57.

Grodstein F, Manson JE, Stampfer MJ. Hormone therapy and coronary heart disease: the role of time since menopause and age at hormone initiation. *J Women's Health* 2006; **15**: 35–44.

Hsia J, Langer RD, Manson JE *et al.* Conjugated equine estrogens and coronary heart disease. The Women's Health Initiative. *Arch Intern Med* 2006; **166**: 357–65.

Maclennan A, Broadbent J, Lester S, Moore V. Oral oestrogen and combined oestrogen/progestogen therapy versus placebo for hot flushes. *Cochrane Database Syst Rev* 2004; **(4)**: CD002978.

Million Women Study Collaborators. Breast cancer and hormone-replacement therapy in the Million Women Study. *Lancet* 2003; **362**: 419–27.

Royal College of Obstetricians and Gynaecologists. *Hormone Replacement Therapy and Venous Thromboembolism.* London: Royal College of Obstetricians and Gynaecologists, 2004.

The Women's Health Initiative Steering Committee. Effects of conjugated equine estrogen in postmenopausal women with hysterectomy: the Women's Health Initiative randomized controlled trial. *JAMA* 2004; **291**: 1701–12.

Writing Group for the Women's Health Initiative Investigators. Risks and benefits of estrogen plus progestin in healthy postmenopausal women: principal results from the Women's Health Initiative randomized controlled trial. *JAMA* 2002; **288**: 321–33.

Websites

British Menopause Society:
   www.the-bms.org (last accessed 6 March 2006).
Cancer Research UK:
   www.cancerresearchuk.org (last accessed 6 March 2006).
National Institute of Health:
   www.consensus.nih.gov (last accessed 6 March 2006).

9 Alternatives to oestrogen for treating menopause symptoms and osteoporosis

Reducing vasomotor symptoms (eg hot flushes)
Reducing vaginal changes
Preventing and treating osteoporosis (brittle bones)
Sources of information

Women who do not want, or who are unable, to take *oestrogen* can consider other options to treat their symptoms and prevent the long-term effects of the menopause.

Reducing vasomotor symptoms (eg hot flushes)

Progestogens such as norethisterone 5 mg/day or *megestrol acetate* 40 mg/day can help to control hot flushes and night sweats. At this dose, norethisterone may also protect the bones a little, but there is no information about whether or not megestrol acetate does the same. However, both these hormones in the doses stated above increase the risk of deep blood clots (*venous thromboembolism*).

Clonidine is licensed for treating hot flushes, but it is of limited use and may cause unpleasant side-effects.

Selective serotonin reuptake inhibitors (SSRIs) are a group of drugs, including Prozac, that are used to treat depression, but they have been shown to reduce hot flushes in short-term studies. They may therefore be useful for women who cannot take oestrogen, such as those who have had breast cancer. However, the long-term benefits of SSRIs are less clear, and there are concerns about safety and problems linked with stopping treatment.

The beta blocker propranolol (widely used to treat high blood pressure) was once recommended for women with hot flushes, but it should not be used because studies of its effects have produced conflicting results.

Reducing vaginal changes

Lubricants and moisturizers are available without prescription. Simple lubricants can help reduce vaginal dryness and prevent discomfort during sex. However, the effect is short lived. Longer acting 'bioadhesive' moisturizers are now available, and one is available on prescription in the UK.

Preventing and treating osteoporosis (brittle bones)

Drug treatments

Bone strength depends on the rate at which new bone is created and the rate at which old bone is destroyed. The removal of old bone is termed resorption. Most medicines designed to prevent or treat *osteoporosis* act by reducing bone resorption (Box 9.1). These treatments have mainly been studied in postmenopausal women who already have osteoporosis or who are at high risk of developing it. Few trials have been done on perimenopausal women or those with an early menopause. In addition, few trials last long enough to provide information about effects of more than 10 years of treatment.

Bisphosphonates
Bone consists of a honeycomb-like framework onto which minerals, such as calcium, are deposited. Bones lose density when these minerals are no longer deposited or through an active process of breakdown called resorption. *Bisphosphonates* are taken up at sites where the bone minerals are deposited and form stable compounds that resist breakdown.

Bisphosphonates are not easily absorbed from the gut, especially if it contains food, and so they should always be taken on an empty stomach. However, they may occasionally irritate the gut and cause symptoms of indigestion. These symptoms stop quickly if you stop taking the bisphosphonate. Gut irritation is also less of a problem with treatments that are taken weekly or monthly rather than daily.

Box 9.1

Treatment for osteoporosis

Bisphosphonates
- Alendronate
- Risedronate
- Ibandronate
- Etidronate

Selective oestrogen receptor modulators (SERMS)
- Raloxifene

Parathyroid hormone
Strontium ranelate
Calcitriol
Calcitonin

Several different bisphosphonates are available. Etidronate, alendronate, risedronate and ibandronate are the ones most often used to prevent and treat osteoporosis.

Alendronate has been shown to reduce fractures of both the spine and hip by half in randomized trials. Several studies have also shown that it maintains and increases the density (BMD) of the hip and spine in postmenopausal women. Unlike etidronate (see below), it may be taken every day or once weekly. The greatest increase is seen in the first year, but BMD continues to increase up to at least 10 years of treatment. Bone mass is preserved for at least two years after treatment is stopped.

Risedronate has been shown to reduce fractures of the spine and other fractures in randomized trials. This effect continues after at least seven years of treatment. Risedronate may be taken daily or weekly.

Ibandronate has been shown to reduce fractures of the spine, but not other types of fracture, by 50% in randomized trials of postmenopausal women. It was introduced in 2005 and may be used to treat or prevent osteoporosis. Ibandronate may be taken daily or monthly.

Etidronate was the first bisphosphonate to be developed. There is solid evidence that it can prevent fractures of the spine, but less strong indications that it also prevents hip fractures. Usually, etidronate is taken for 14 of every 90 days, and calcium is taken for the other 76 days. It may seem strange, but taking etidronate continuously rather than in 14-day sessions actually increases bone loss.

How long should bisphosphonates be taken?
This question is still being debated. It is possible that continuous, long-term use of bisphosphonates may actually damage the bone, although shorter or periodic treatment is definitely beneficial. Some doctors therefore recommend a two-year 'holiday' after alendronate has been taken for five years.

Which bisphosphonate is best?
Studies have compared alendronate with risedronate, but they measured bone density rather than risk of fracture, so the results are hard to interpret. Weekly or monthly preparations may cause fewer gut problems than daily preparations, and some women find them more convenient.

Selective oestrogen receptor modulators (SERMS)
The hormone oestrogen acts by binding to cellular receptors. Different receptors occur on different types of cell. Some substances therefore affect the oestrogen receptors on some cells but not others. Some chemicals even have opposite effects in different tissues and organs. These are called selective

oestrogen receptor modulators, or SERMs (the acronym refers to the American spelling, which is estrogen). One of the first SERMs was tamoxifen, which is widely used to treat breast cancer but is not recommended for the treatment or prevention of osteoporosis.

Raloxifene was the first SERM to be licensed to prevent fractures of the spine caused by osteoporosis. In women who already have osteoporosis, raloxifene can reduce spine fractures by between one-third and one-half, depending on the dose, but it does not seem to reduce the risk of fractures in other bones, such as the hip.

Raloxifene can cause short-term side-effects such as hot flushes and calf cramps. It does not treat the symptoms of the menopause and is therefore not suitable for women with hot flushes. Like hormone replacement therapy (*HRT*), it increases the risk of deep blood clots (VTE) (see Chapter 5). However, it protects the bone without affecting the womb lining (*endometrium*) or the breast. It therefore does not cause any bleeding or breast tenderness. It also reduces the risk of breast cancer if taken long term in women with osteoporosis. Raloxifene also reduces cholesterol levels and may prevent heart disease. At higher doses, it has been shown to reduce memory problems and *dementia* in postmenopausal women with osteoporosis.

Raloxifene is probably most useful for women aged 60–75 years who are at high risk of fractures of the spine but who cannot, or prefer not to, take HRT.

Parathyroid hormone

This hormone is produced by four small glands found in the neck, near the *thyroid*. People whose *parathyroid glands* are overactive (a condition called hyperparathyroidism) may experience bone loss, but if parathyroid hormone is taken in short pulses, it seems to have the opposite effect. A study of more than 1600 postmenopausal women with osteoporosis showed that parathyroid hormone led to a significant decrease in the risk of fractures in the spine. It is used in cases of severe osteoporosis and is given by a daily injection. The benefits may be even greater if parathyroid hormone is taken together with HRT.

Strontium ranelate

Strontium is a naturally occurring element that is similar to calcium. It was used widely in the 1950s but fell out of favour because of harmful effects on bone metabolism. However, these problems may have been due to calcium-deficient diets or the use of the wrong dose. Randomized controlled trials have shown that strontium can reduce the risk of fractures of the spine and hip. It is taken as a powder that is dissolved in water and should be taken daily at least two hours after food. It occasionally causes mild nausea and diarrhoea.

Calcitriol
This is a natural substance formed in the body by the breakdown of vitamin D. It helps calcium to be absorbed from food and also has direct effects on bone cells. People who take *calcitriol* need to have their calcium levels checked frequently. Studies of calcitriol have not produced clear results – often because they did not involve enough patients. The largest study involved more than 600 postmenopausal women. Half of them took calcitriol and the other half took only calcium. The women who took only calcium had more new fractures during the study than before, while those taking calcitriol had no change in the rate of fractures. The finding that women who took calcium had an increased fracture rate is unexpected and hard to explain.

Calcitonin
Calcitonin controls the balance between bone formation and breakdown. It currently cannot be taken by mouth, but it is available as an injection or nasal spray. Injections are expensive, often cause side-effects such as sickness, diarrhoea and hot flushes and may cause allergic reactions. Nasal calcitonin has been shown to reduce fractures of the spine and reduce the pain caused by them. It may also be helpful after surgery for hip fracture. An oral form is being developed.

Future developments
Statins are a class of drug used to lower cholesterol. It has been suggested that statins might reduce the risk of fractures. This has not yet been tested in randomized trials. Although fluoride is known to strengthen teeth, its use in osteoporosis has not been clearly shown, so it is not recommended. Future developments include bisphosphonates that can be taken just once a year, new SERMs and new types of drugs that affect bone remodelling.

Other approaches to osteoporosis

Calcium and vitamin D
Whatever treatment is used to prevent or treat osteoporosis, it is important that women get enough calcium and vitamin D – either from food or in supplements. British women, especially the elderly, often lack vitamin D. Most of our vitamin D comes from the action of sunlight on the skin. Good dietary sources include oily fish, fortified cereals and soft spreads such as margarines.

Vitamin D is produced by the skin when it is exposed to sunlight. Because of Britain's northerly position, the skin only produces vitamin D in the summer, and our national diet lacks sufficient vitamin D to make up for this. In other countries, even those with more sunshine, such as the United States, dairy products are fortified with vitamin D.

The current recommended daily dose of calcium in the UK is 700 mg. However, most studies show that women need about 1.5 g (ie more than twice the recommended amount) to keep their bones healthy after the menopause if they are not taking HRT. A lower dose of 1.0 g is enough for women who are using HRT.

Women who do not want, or who are unable, to take calcium supplements should be careful to include calcium-rich foods in their diet. Table 9.1 shows the calcium content of some foods.

Studies of calcium and vitamin D have been contradictory. This may be because results depend on the type of people who enter the study. For example, people in residential homes may be more frail or have lower intakes of calcium and vitamin D from food than people living independently.

Table 9.1

Calcium content of some foods

Food	Calcium content (mg)
Full-fat milk (250 ml)	295
Semi-skimmed milk (250 ml)	300
Skimmed milk (250 ml)	305
Low-fat yogurt (100 g)	150
Cheddar cheese (50 g)	360
Boiled spinach (100 g)	159
Brazil nuts (100 g)	170
Tinned salmon (100 g)	93
Tofu (100 g)	480

Evidence about calcium

Combined results of 15 studies involving more than 1800 people show that calcium taken for at least two years reduces the rates of bone loss and increases bone density compared with no or dummy treatment (*placebo*). However, it was not clear whether or not this translated into a meaningful reduction in the risk of fractures. Although calcium probably slows the rate of bone loss after the menopause, it cannot make weak bones stronger.

Evidence about vitamin D

Combined results of 12 studies involving more than 19,000 people suggest that 700–800 international units per day of vitamin D reduces the risk of hip or other fractures by about one-quarter (25%) compared with calcium or placebo. Lower doses (400 international units per day) are less effective.

Evidence about calcium plus vitamin D

Early studies suggested that taking calcium and vitamin D supplements could reduce the risk of hip fractures. However, more recent studies in women living in the community or in those who already have osteoporosis have been less convincing. In fact the randomized WHI study undertaken in the United States found no reduction of fracture and a small increase in kidney stones.

Sources of information

Journal articles

Bischoff-Ferrari HA, Willett WC, Wong JB *et al*. Fracture prevention with vitamin D supplementation: a meta-analysis of randomized controlled trials. *JAMA* 2005; **293**: 2257–64.

Grant AM, Avenell A, Campbell MK *et al*. Oral vitamin D3 and calcium for secondary prevention of low-trauma fractures in elderly people (Randomised Evaluation of Calcium Or vitamin D, RECORD): a randomised placebo-controlled trial. *Lancet* 2005; **365**: 1621–8.

Jackson RD, LaCroix AZ, Gass M *et al*; Women's Health Initiative Investigators. Calcium plus vitamin D supplementation and the risk of fractures. *N Engl J Med* 2006; **354**: 669–83.

McClung MR, Lewiecki EM, Cohen SB *et al*; AMG 162 Bone Loss Study Group. Denosumab in postmenopausal women with low bone mineral density. *N Engl J Med* 2006; **354**: 821–31.

Nieves JW. Osteoporosis: the role of micronutrients. *Am J Clin Nutr* 2005; **81**: 1232S–9S.

Pandya KJ, Morrow GR, Roscoe JA *et al*. Gabapentin for hot flashes in 420 women with breast cancer: a randomised double-blind placebo-controlled trial. *Lancet* 2005; **366**: 818–24.

Porthouse J, Cockayne S, King C *et al*. Randomised controlled trial of calcium and supplementation with cholecalciferol (vitamin D3) for prevention of fractures in primary care. *BMJ* 2005; **330**: 1003–6.

Reginster JY, Seeman E, De Vernejoul MC *et al*. Strontium ranelate reduces the risk of nonvertebral fractures in postmenopausal women with osteoporosis: Treatment of Peripheral Osteoporosis (TROPOS) Study. *J Clin Endocrinol Metab* 2005; **90**: 2816–22.

Reginster JY, Wilson KM, Dumont E *et al*. Monthly oral ibandronate is well tolerated and efficacious in postmenopausal women: results from the monthly oral pilot study. *J Clin Endocrinol Metab* 2005; **90**: 5018–24.

Ruggiero SL, Mehrotra B, Rosenberg TJ, Engroff SL. Osteonecrosis of the jaws associated with the use of bisphosphonates: a review of 63 cases. *J Oral Maxillofac Surg* 2004; **62**: 527–34.

Shea B, Wells G, Cranney A *et al*. Calcium supplementation on bone loss in postmenopausal women. *Cochrane Database Syst Rev* 2004; (1): CD004526.

Siris ES, Harris ST, Eastell R *et al*. Skeletal effects of raloxifene after 8 years: results from the Continuing Outcomes Relevant to Evista (CORE) Study. *J Bone Miner Res* 2005; **20**: 1514–24.

Suvanto-Luukkonen E, Koivunen R, Sundstrom H *et al.* Citalopram and fluoxetine in the treatment of postmenopausal symptoms: a prospective, randomized, 9-month, placebo-controlled, double-blind study. *Menopause* 2005; **12:** 18–26.

Book

Rees M, Mander T. *Managing the Menopause without Oestrogen.* London: Royal Society of Medicine Press, 2004.

Websites

National Osteoporosis Foundation:
    www.nof.org (last accessed 6 March 2006).
National Osteoporosis Society:
    www.nos.org.uk (last accessed 6 March 2006).

10 Diet, exercise and hip protectors

Diet
Exercise
Hip protectors
Sources of information

Diet and regular exercise are important in protecting against heart disease and brittle bones (*osteoporosis*). Regular physical activity may also reduce symptoms of the menopause, such as hot flushes and mood changes. Weight-bearing and muscle-strengthening exercises help maintain bone mass, but the effects wear off when exercise is stopped. Although improving your diet and taking more exercise when you reach the menopause can be helpful, they cannot make up for an unhealthy lifestyle up to that point.

Diet

A healthy diet aims to prevent you becoming either too fat or too thin and should also provide the vitamins and minerals your body needs. Eating the right type of foods may also help prevent diseases such as heart attacks and cancer.

Fat

Avoiding saturated fats can reduce the risk of heart disease. Simple ways of reducing your saturated fat intake are to replace butter with a low-fat spread or margarine, use skimmed or semi-skimmed milk instead of full-fat milk and choose lean cuts of meat. The type of fats found in oily fish (called long-chain omega 3 fatty acids) may also improve *cardiovascular* health and reduce the risk of diabetes. These fats are found in fish such as mackerel, herrings and sardines. However the WHI randomized trial found reducing total fat intake did not reduce the risk of *coronary* heart disease or stroke. This suggests that altering the types of fat in the diet such as reducing saturated fats is more important.

Carbohydrate

Sugars such as sucrose and glucose provide energy but no other nutrients. Sugary foods may also cause diabetes. A balanced diet should contain plenty of wholegrain cereals and starchy vegetables that contain fibre and useful vitamins, as well as providing energy. Try to eat wholegrain breakfast cereals, brown bread and pasta rather than more refined carbohydrates (sugary cereals, white bread and ordinary pasta). Sugar, jam, puddings and sweets may be eaten in moderation.

Protein

Make sure your diet contains enough protein. This can come from meat, dairy products, nuts and pulses (beans and lentils). Older people may actually need more protein than younger adults, although not enough research has been done in this area. In patients who are ill, are recovering from surgery or have infections or pressure ulcers, the body needs more protein than usual. Lack of protein may lead to reduced muscle mass, lowered resistance to diseases and poor wound healing.

Vitamins and minerals

See Chapter 9 for information about calcium and vitamin D.

Several studies have suggested that people who eat a lot of fruit and vegetables have a lower risk of many illnesses. This may be because fruit and vegetables contain a number of chemicals called antioxidants, such as vitamins E and C. Antioxidants protect against damage from free radicals, which are substances produced normally by the body but which may be linked with disease and ageing. However, no studies have shown that taking supplements of a single antioxidant can improve health. In fact, taking vitamin E may increase the risk of heart failure in women with heart disease, and high doses of vitamin C seem to increase the risk of heart disease in postmenopausal women with diabetes.

You should try to eat at least five portions of fruit or vegetables per day. Surveys suggest that most women aged 50–64 years eat less than this. Eating lots of types of fruits and vegetables (not the same ones every time) probably brings the greatest benefits.

Vitamin and mineral supplements may be helpful if your diet is lacking these substances, but they can be harmful, especially at high doses. Safe upper limits, recommended by the UK Food Standards Agency, are shown in Table 10.1.

Functional foods

This term refers to foods thought to carry a health benefit beyond simple nutrition.

Table 10.1

Safe upper levels for intake of selected antioxidants. Source: Expert Group on Vitamins and Minerals, Food Standards Agency (2003)

Nutrient	Safe upper level (per day)
Beta-carotene	9 mg
Selenium	0.45 mg
Vitamin E	800 IU (540 mg d-α-tocopherol equivalents/day)
Vitamin C	Insufficient evidence

Probiotics

These are foods that contain live micro-organisms that may improve the natural balance of such organisms in your body. Several bio-yoghurts, drinks and cereals contain bacteria belonging to the *Lactobacillus* and *Bifidobacterium* groups. These can improve gut conditions such as irritable bowel syndrome and may benefit other conditions such as thrush (candidiasis) and other infections.

Prebiotics

These foods, although they do not contain helpful micro-organisms, are thought to encourage them. Prebiotics are types of sugars that cannot be digested and cannot be metabolized by non-probiotic gut flora such as *Bacteroides* species and *Escherichia coli*. Prebiotics are available naturally in breast milk and in certain vegetables (for example, Jerusalem artichokes and onions). They may affect the body's ability to absorb calcium.

Synbiotics

These products contain both probiotic and prebiotic ingredients. They are therefore designed to introduce healthy micro-organisms to the body and to help them become established. Few clinical studies of such products have been performed.

Nutraceuticals

Nutraceuticals are natural components of foods (such as *phytoestrogens*) and are released during digestion in the gut. They are thought to have a direct effect on health (see Chapter 11 for more details).

Fibre

Dietary fibre consists of structures found in plants, which cannot be broken down by the gut. The presence of fibre in the diet improves the passage of food through the gut and may also lower cholesterol and improve the control of blood sugar. One reason why experts recommend that everybody should eat at least five portions of fruit or vegetables per day is that these contain valuable fibre. A diet high in fibre seems to reduce the risk of developing various diseases, including heart disease and certain types of cancer, but the evidence is conflicting.

The Mediterranean diet

Several studies have suggested that eating a typical Mediterranean diet can increase life expectancy and reduce the risk of several serious diseases (Table 10.2).

Table 10.2

Features of the Mediterranean diet

Food group	Example/type	Amount of food group in Mediterranean diet
Vegetables and pulses (lentils)		High
Fruit		High
Cereals	Mostly unrefined	High
Unsaturated fats	Olive oil	High
Fish		Moderate to high
Dairy products	Cheese and yoghurt	Low to moderate
Meat		Low
Saturated fats		Low
Alcohol	Mostly as wine	Modest

Exercise

For postmenopausal women, regular physical activity has been shown to reduce the risk of fractures, heart disease, diabetes and *dementia*. Menopause symptoms such as hot flushes, insomnia, incontinence and depression may also be improved by exercise. Exercise can be grouped into types that improve endurance (aerobic), strength (resistance) or balance (such as Tai Chi).

Exercise and osteoporosis

The benefits of exercise in preventing brittle bones and fractures are well known. However, it is not so clear what kind of exercise you need to take, or for how long, to get the benefits. Brisk walking about three times per week seems to increase the strength of the spine and hips. Weight-bearing exercise seems only to increase the strength of the spine (not the hips). Women who already have osteoporosis can also be helped by exercise. The main benefits come from increased wellbeing, muscle strength and balance rather than increased bone mass. However, people with osteoporosis need to exercise carefully to avoid falls.

Exercise and coronary heart disease

Physical activity increases oxygen delivery around the body and improves the heart and blood vessels. Exercise can also improve the *lipid* profile, increasing the amounts of 'good' (high-density lipoprotein) cholesterol. It may also prevent narrowing of the arteries (*atherosclerosis*). Once again, it is not yet clear how much you need to exercise to get these benefits. However, recent evidence suggests that low-impact exercise, such as walking, may be just as healthy as more vigorous activities and also carries less risk of injury.

Exercise and urinary incontinence

Pelvic floor exercises may be helpful for women with stress incontinence. However, the effects on urgency are less clear, and most information has come from premenopausal women, so more information is required.

Hip protectors

Padded hip protectors have been recommended to prevent hip fractures in elderly women. (Figure 10.1). However, the protectors are not particularly

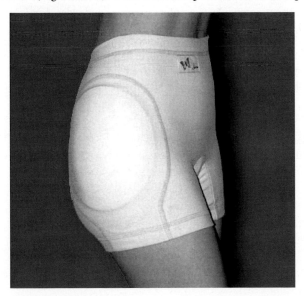

Figure 10.1 Hip protectors. Reprinted with permission from HipSaver Inc.,Canton, MA, USA

attractive, are uncomfortable in hot weather and may be difficult to fit. A randomized trial of women older than 70 years who lived in the community in the UK found no benefit from hip protectors. Also their effectiveness for women living in residential homes is uncertain.

Sources of information

Journal articles

Birks YF, Porthouse J, Addie C *et al.* Randomized controlled trial of hip protectors among women living in the community. *Osteoporos Int* 2004; **15**: 701–6.

Din JN, Newby DE, Flapan AD. Omega 3 fatty acids and cardiovascular disease – fishing for a natural treatment. *BMJ* 2004; **328**: 30–5.

Hamilton-Miller JM. Probiotics and prebiotics in the elderly. *Postgrad Med J* 2004; **80**: 447–51.

Howard BV, Van Horn L, Hsia J *et al.* Low-fat dietary pattern and risk of cardiovascular disease: The Women's Health Initiative Randomized Controlled Dietary Modification Trial. *JAMA* 2006; **295**: 655–66.

Kennedy E, Meyers L. Dietary Reference Intakes: development and uses for assessment of micronutrient status of women – a global perspective. *Am J Clin Nutr* 2005; **81**: 1194S-7S.

Knoops KT, de Groot LC, Kromhout D *et al.* Mediterranean diet, lifestyle factors, and 10-year mortality in elderly European men and women: the HALE project. *JAMA* 2004; **292**: 1433–9.

Larson EB, Wang L, Bowen JD *et al.* Exercise is associated with reduced risk for incident dementia among persons 65 years of age and older. *Ann Intern Med* 2006; **144**: 73–81.

Parker MJ, Gillespie WJ, Gillespie LD. Effectiveness of hip protectors for preventing hip fractures in elderly people: systematic review. *BMJ* 2006; **332**: 571–4.

Qin L, Choy W, Leung K *et al.* Beneficial effects of regular Tai Chi exercise on musculoskeletal system. *J Bone Miner Metab* 2005; **23**: 186–90.

Website

Food Standard Agency:
www.food.gov.uk (last accessed 6 March 2006).

11 Alternative and complementary therapies

Phytoestrogens
Herbalism
Homeopathy
Dehydroepiandrosterone
Progesterone transdermal creams
Acupuncture
Reflexology
Magnets
Sources of information

Little scientific evidence shows that complementary and alternative therapies can help menopausal symptoms or provide the same benefits as hormone replacement therapy (*HRT*). Yet many women use them, believing them to be safer and 'more natural' than products prescribed by their doctor. Concerns about the safety of *oestrogen*-based HRT have also increased since the publication of the Women's Health Initiative study and the Million Women Study. In the UK, more than one in 10 adults visit a therapist each year, and nearly half are taking a food supplement. The choice of treatments is confusing and, unlike conventional medicines, not much is known about their safety or side-effects or how they may interact with other therapies. Some herbal preparations may contain oestrogen-like substances, which is a concern for women with hormone-dependent diseases, such as breast cancer. There is also concern about the lack of strict quality controls in the production of these therapies.

Phytoestrogens

Phytoestrogens are plant substances that have effects similar to those of oestrogens. Preparations vary from enriched foods such as bread or drinks (soy milk) to more concentrated tablets. The most important groups are called isoflavones and lignans. The major isoflavones are genistein and daidzein. The major lignans are enterolactone and enterodiol.

Isoflavones are found in soybeans, chick peas, red clover and probably other legumes (beans and peas). Oil seeds, such as flaxseed, are rich in lignans, and they are also found in cereal bran, whole cereals, vegetables, legumes and fruit.

Interest in phytoestrogens has been stimulated by the observation that women in countries where the diet is rich in isoflavones, such as Japan, seem to have lower rates of menopausal symptoms; heart disease; *osteoporosis*; and cancers of the breast, large intestine (colon), womb lining (*endometrium*) and *ovary*. But it is not straightforward to translate these observations into helpful recommendations for women in other countries, as other factors in the Japanese diet or genetic differences between the populations might be involved. Evidence from randomized *placebo*-controlled trials in Western women of the effects of soy and red clover on menopause symptoms is inconsistent. The effects of such compounds on the blood vessels, brain and womb are also unclear.

Phytoestrogens and the synthetic isoflavone ipriflavone may help maintain bone mass, but the evidence is conflicting. Some short-term studies suggest a beneficial effect, but the best dose is not yet known. There are also concerns about side-effects; in particular, ipriflavone may cause loss of white blood cells (lymphocytopenia) in a significant number of women.

Further well-designed research is needed to discover whether or not phytoestrogen supplements are effective and safe treatments for women with menopausal symptoms.

Herbalism

Some herbs (such as ginseng) have strong oestrogenic properties (ie they act in the same way as oestrogen), so women who cannot take oestrogen should be very careful when trying herbal treatments. Herbal remedies may also alter the effects of treatments prescribed by your doctor or cause dangerous side-effects. They can interact with blood-thinning drugs such as warfarin, antidepressants, drugs used for epilepsy and general anaesthetics. They can either increase or reduce the effects of prescribed treatments. For example, ginkgo can cause bleeding when taken with *warfarin* or aspirin, high blood pressure when taken with some diuretics (water tablets) and even coma when taken with the antidepressant trazodone. St John's wort reduces the levels, and therefore the activity, of several drugs. There have been cases in which reduced concentrations of drugs have led to organ rejection after transplants and unplanned pregnancies in women taking St John's wort while using oral contraceptives.

Another problem with herbal remedies and supplements is that there is little control over their quality, and it is often impossible to know exactly what they contain. Some contain high levels of chemicals such as pesticides, arsenic, lead and mercury. Cases of kidney failure, liver failure and even cancer have been linked to herbal treatments. A European Union Directive was implemented in the UK in October 2005, which will hopefully help.

If you are taking a herbal treatment, you must tell your doctor before they prescribe a medicine for you.

Box 11.1 summarizes the herbs used by menopausal women.

Box 11.1

Herbs used by menopausal women

Actaea racemosa (*black cohosh*)
Piper methysticum (*kava kava*)
Oenothera bienis (*evening primrose*)
Angelica sinensis (*dong quai*)
Ginkgo biloba (*gingko*)
Panax ginseng (*ginseng*)
Others, such as wild yam cream, St John's wort, Agnus castus (*chasteberry*), liquorice root and Valerian root

---

Black cohosh (Actaea racemosa, *formerly called* Cimicifuga racemosa)

This is a herbaceous plant from North America that is widely used to treat symptoms of the menopause. Laboratory studies show that it contains substances that bind to oestrogen receptors, but we do not know if this explains its effects. Results from studies that compared black cohosh with placebo (dummy treatment) or HRT are promising, but little is known about its long-term safety.

Kava kava (Piper methysticum)

This has been used for thousands of years in the South Pacific for recreational and medical purposes. Data pooled from a number of studies suggested it may reduce anxiety, but its effects on menopause symptoms are not clear. However, concern about liver damage has led many European authorities to ban kava kava.

Oil of evening primrose (Oenothera biennis)

This oil contains gamma-linolenic acid. One small placebo-controlled randomized trial found it had no effect on hot flushes.

Dong quai (Angelica sinensis)

This is a perennial plant found in southwest China and used in traditional Chinese medicine. A randomized trial found that it had no more effect on menopausal symptoms than placebo (dummy treatment). It can interact with warfarin and cause the skin to become very sensitive to sunlight.

Gingko (Gingko biloba)

Many women use gingko, but little evidence shows that it improves menopausal symptoms.

Ginseng (Panax ginseng)

This grows in Korea and China and is widely used in eastern Asia. A randomized trial found that it had no more effect on menopausal symptoms than placebo (dummy treatment). Cases of vaginal bleeding and breast pain have been linked with ginseng use. This is most likely to be the result of its oestrogenic effects. It can interact with warfarin (used to thin blood), phenelzine (an antidepressant) and alcohol.

Ginseng is a popular therapy for postmenopausal women. It has little effect on hot flushes, but it may improve depression and wellbeing.

Others

Wild yam cream, St John's wort, chasteberry (*Agnus castus*), liquorice root and Valerian root are also popular, but there is no evidence that they have any effect on menopausal symptoms. Claims have been made that steroids in yams can be converted to *progesterone* in the human body, but this is biochemically impossible.

Homeopathy

The theory of homeopathy was developed by Samuel Hahnemann – an 18th century German doctor. He believed that patients with particular signs and symptoms can be cured if given a drug that produces the same effects in a healthy person. He found that the effects were strongest when the substance was highly diluted and shaken vigorously. However, the mechanisms that might explain a biological response to solutions that may not even contain one molecule of the active substance are not clear. Results from individual cases, observational studies and a small number of randomized trials are encouraging, but more research is needed.

Dehydroepiandrosterone

Dehydroepiandrosterone (DHEA) is a naturally occurring steroid produced by cells around the kidneys (called the *adrenal* glands). Blood levels of DHEA drop dramatically with age. This had led to suggestions that the effects of ageing can be counteracted by DHEA 'replacement therapy'. It is increasingly being used in the USA, where it is classed as a food supplement, for its supposed anti-ageing effects. Some studies have shown benefits on the skeleton, thought processes (cognition), wellbeing and the vagina. The short-term effects of taking DHEA are still controversial, and possible harmful effects of long-term use are, as yet, unknown.

Progesterone transdermal creams

Several progesterone gels and creams are available. One gel has been licensed in Europe for local use on the breast but not for *systemic* treatment. The amount of progesterone in the different products ranges from 0.17 to 64 mg per gram of product. There is not enough evidence to show that progesterone applied to the skin can reduce *vasomotor* symptoms (hot flushes) or prevent osteoporosis (brittle bones).

Women who have not had a *hysterectomy* are at increased risk of growths and cancer of the womb lining (endometrium) if they take oestrogen alone (see Chapter 5). Adding a progestogen or progesterone reduces this risk. However, the available evidence suggests that progesterone creams do not provide enough progesterone to offer protection. They should therefore **not** be used in order to protect the womb lining from the effects of oestrogen.

Acupuncture

This is based on traditional Chinese medicine and uses needles to stimulate special points on the body. A randomized controlled trial of electro-acupuncture showed no benefit for symptoms of the menopause (Figure 11.1).

Reflexology

Reflexology is based on the theory that areas on the feet correspond to, and therefore can affect, other parts of the body (Figure 11.2). Few studies have looked at reflexology for menopausal complaints. Only one randomized trial has been published so far, and it showed no improvement in vasomotor symptoms (such as hot flushes). The benefits of reflexology are therefore uncertain.

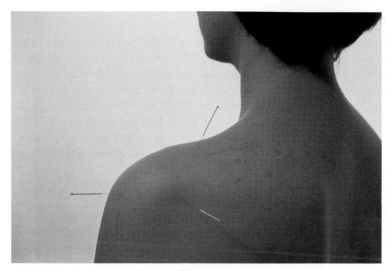

Figure 11.1 Acupuncture needles. Courtesy of British Acupuncture Council

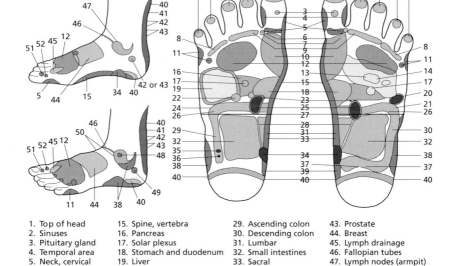

1. Top of head	15. Spine, vertebra	29. Ascending colon	43. Prostate
2. Sinuses	16. Pancreas	30. Descending colon	44. Breast
3. Pituitary gland	17. Solar plexus	31. Lumbar	45. Lymph drainage
4. Temporal area	18. Stomach and duodenum	32. Small intestines	46. Fallopian tubes
5. Neck, cervical	19. Liver	33. Sacral	47. Lymph nodes (armpit)
6. Upper lymph area	20. Spleen	34. Bladder	48. Sacro-iliac joint
7. Parathyroid gland	21. Splenic fixture	35. Ilio-caecal valve	49. Ovary or testicle
8. Ears	22. Gall bladder	36. Appendix	50. Lymph nodes (groin)
9. Eyes	23. Adrenal glands	37. Sigmoid flexure	51. Maxilla/submaxilla (jaw)
10. Thyroid glands	24. Hepatic flexure	38. Hip and lower back	52. Tonsils
11. Shoulder	25. Kidneys	39. Coccyx	
12. Lungs and bronchi	26. Transverse colon	40. Sciatic area	
13. Heart area	27. Waist	41. Rectum	
14. Heart	28. Ureters	42. Uterus	

Figure 11.2 Reflexology chart

Magnets

There is no known mechanism of action for magnet therapies for the treatment of hot flushes. Little is known about its effect on menopausal symptoms. One small study has shown no benefit.

Sources of information

Journal articles

Balk E, Chung M, Chew P et al. Effects of soy on health outcomes. *Evid Rep Technol Assess (Summ)* 2005; **126**: 1–8.

Carpenter JS, Neal JG. Other complementary and alternative medicine modalities: acupuncture, magnets, reflexology, and homeopathy. *Am J Med* 2005; **118** (12 Suppl 2): 109–17.

Dog TL. Menopause: a review of botanical dietary supplements. *Am J Med* 2005; **118** (12 Suppl 2): 98–108.

Ernst E. The efficacy of herbal medicine – an overview. *Fundam Clin Pharmacol* 2005; **19**: 405–9.

Hu Z, Yang X, Ho PC et al. Herb-drug interactions: a literature review. *Drugs* 2005; **65**: 1239–82.

Jutte R, Riley D. A review of the use and role of low potencies in homeopathy. *Complement Ther Med* 2005; **13**: 291–6.

Sacks FM, Lichtenstein A, Van Horn L et al. Soy protein, isoflavones, and cardiovascular health. An American Heart Association Science Advisory for Professionals from the Nutrition Committee. *Circulation* 2006; **113**: 1034–44.

Book

Rees M, Mander T. *Managing the Menopause without Oestrogen*. London: Royal Society of Medicine Press, 2004.

Websites

American Cancer Society (ACS), *Complementary and alternative therapies*:
www.cancer.org/docroot (last accessed 6 April 2006).

BBC Health:
www.bbc.co.uk/health (last accessed 6 April 2006).

Medicines and Healthcare Products Regulatory Agency (MHRA), Traditional Herbal Medicines Registration Scheme:
www.mhra.gov.uk/ (last accessed 6 April 2006).

National Center for Complementary and Alternative Medicine, National Institutes of Health:
http://nccam.nih.gov/ (last accessed 6 April 2006).

Office of Dietary Supplements (home page):
http://dietary-supplements.info.nih.gov/ (last accessed 6 April 2006).

12 Early (premature) menopause

As the normal age for menopause varies between different women, defining an early menopause is a matter of judgement. In the developed world, most doctors consider that a woman whose periods stop before she is aged 45 years fits the category of an early menopause. However, estimates of the average age at menopause in developing countries may not always be accurate. Therefore, the age of 40 years is used frequently as an arbitrary limit below which the menopause is said to be premature.

The condition is not uncommon: about one in a hundred (1%) of women younger than 40 years go through the menopause and one in a thousand (0.1%) women younger than 30 years.

Doctors describe naturally occurring menopause as primary and menopause due to surgery, radiotherapy or chemotherapy as secondary (Box 12.1).

Box 12.1

Causes of ovarian failure

Primary
- Chromosome abnormalities
- Enzyme deficiencies
- Autoimmune diseases

Secondary
- Chemotherapy and radiotherapy
- Surgery
- Infection

Primary premature ovarian failure

Primary premature ovarian failure (POF) means the woman's ovaries stop working. It is usually not possible to tell why this happens. Although lack of periods usually means the ovaries have stopped producing eggs, they sometimes start up again, so women with this condition are not always infertile and need to consider contraception.

Chromosome abnormalities

One possible cause of primary POF is an abnormality on one of the chromosomes. For example, women with the 'Fragile X' mutation are 10 times more likely to have POF than those without. Women with Down's syndrome (which is caused by having one extra chromosome) and Turner syndrome (which is caused by having only one X chromosome rather than the normal pair) also have an early menopause.

Enzyme deficiencies

Conditions in which the body cannot produce enough of certain enzymes or produces an altered form of an enzyme may be linked with POF. Examples include inherited galactosaemia and deficiencies of the enzymes 17-alpha-hydroxylase and 17,20-desmolase. These affect the ovaries by damaging the eggs and preventing production of *oestrogen*.

Autoimmune diseases

Antibodies are usually produced in response to foreign substances such as bacteria or viruses and are the body's natural defence mechanism. However, in some people, the body produces antibodies that damage its own tissues. This causes autoimmune diseases. Various autoimmune diseases are linked with POF, particularly hypothyroidism (in which the *thyroid* gland does not work properly). About one-quarter of women with POF will have hypothyroidism. Premature ovarian failure is associated with other conditions, including Addison's disease (in which the *adrenal* glands do not work properly) and diabetes mellitus, but only in up to 3% of women with these conditions.

Secondary premature ovarian failure

Various illnesses and medical treatments can also cause POF.

Chemotherapy and radiotherapy

The risk of POF from chemotherapy or radiotherapy depends on the type of treatment given and the age of the patient. Younger women, especially those who have not yet reached puberty, can tolerate stronger chemotherapy and radiotherapy without losing fertility than older women. If you are concerned about the effects of cancer treatment on fertility, you should discuss this with your doctor. In some women, it is possible to remove eggs before treatment and store them for later use.

Radiotherapy may also damage the womb, and women who have had radiotherapy in childhood have a higher rate of pregnancy complications and premature babies.

Surgical menopause

The operation to remove both ovaries (called *bilateral oophorectomy*) causes an immediate menopause. Women who have a surgical menopause often experience marked symptoms (in contrast to some women who pass the natural menopause with few or very minor symptoms).

Hysterectomy without oophorectomy (removal of the womb but not the ovaries)

Women who have a *hysterectomy* (surgery to remove the womb) may have an early menopause – even if the ovaries are not removed. Sometimes this happens straight after the operation, while in other people, the effect is delayed but the menopause is still earlier than normal. Diagnosis can be difficult, as removal of the womb stops the monthly bleeds and not all women have marked symptoms.

Infection

Some infections, notably tuberculosis (TB) and mumps, may cause POF; however, ovarian function returns after mumps in most cases. Other infections that have been linked with POF include malaria and chickenpox (varicella).

Effects of an early menopause

Women who have an early menopause are at increased risk of developing *osteoporosis* and heart disease but at lower risk of getting breast cancer than women whose menopause occurs at the normal time. The risk of heart disease is especially pronounced in smokers.

Possible treatments

Counselling and self-help groups

Women who experience an early menopause before they have been able to have children may find it hard to come to terms with their condition.

Counselling or talking to other women with POF may be helpful. In the UK, the Daisy Network runs special self-help groups for women with POF. There is also the International Premature Ovarian Failure Association (IPOFA).

Hormone replacement therapy (HRT)

Most doctors recommend that women who have an early menopause should take *HRT* until they reach the normal age for natural menopause (which is 52 years). This should not increase the risk of breast cancer above that for women with a normal menopause. No clinical trials have tested the usefulness of alternatives to oestrogen such as *bisphosphonates* or raloxifene in women with an early menopause (see Chapter 9). Some types of contraceptive pill may be used to provide HRT. This may be a more acceptable way of taking oestrogen for young women. In addition, women with POF may need higher doses of oestrogen to control *vasomotor* symptoms (eg hot flushes) than women in their 50s.

Some women, especially those who have had an oophorectomy, continue to have problems with tiredness and loss of interest or pleasure in sex despite using HRT. They may benefit from *testosterone*. Testosterone implants are currently available, and testosterone patches and gels are being developed.

Fertility issues

For women with POF who do not have major chromosome abnormalities, the lifetime chance of becoming pregnant naturally is 5–15%. As yet, no simple test exists to measure fertility in these cases. *In vitro* fertilization (IVF) using donated eggs is a possibility. Success rates with IVF for women with POF are the same as for other women. One study has shown that using eggs donated by a sister gives a lower pregnancy rate than using eggs from an unrelated donor.

Women with Turner syndrome can also have IVF using a donated egg, but the risk of miscarriage is higher in these cases. In addition, women with Turner syndrome have a higher risk of pregnancy complications, such as high blood pressure and pre-eclampsia (toxaemia of pregnancy), so they need to consider the extra risk of a multiple pregnancy if more than one egg is transferred.

Eggs (*oocytes*) may be frozen before a woman has chemotherapy or radiotherapy. Successful pregnancies have been achieved using this method, but the technique is difficult, and success rates are not high. Collecting the eggs requires hormone treatment to stimulate the ovaries. This may not be advisable for women with oestrogen-sensitive tumours. In some cases, if there is time, an embryo may be frozen.

Sources of information

Journal articles

Beerendonk CC, Braat DD. Present and future options for the preservation of fertility in female adolescents with cancer. *Endocr Dev* 2005; **8**: 166–75.

Donnez J, Dolmans MM, Demylle D *et al*. Livebirth after orthotopic transplantation of cryopreserved ovarian tissue. *Lancet* 2004; **364**: 1405–10.

Lutchman Singh K, Davies M, Chatterjee R. Fertility in female cancer survivors: pathophysiology, preservation and the role of ovarian reserve testing. *Hum Reprod Update* 2005; **11**: 69–89.

Nelson LM, Covington SN, Rebar RW. An update: spontaneous premature ovarian failure is not an early menopause. *Fertil Steril* 2005; **83**: 1327–32.

Ossewaarde ME, Bots ML, Verbeek AL *et al*. Age at menopause, cause-specific mortality and total life expectancy. *Epidemiology* 2005; **16**: 556–62.

Rebar RW. Mechanisms of premature menopause. *Endocrinol Metab Clin North Am* 2005; **34**: 923–33.

Sklar C. Maintenance of ovarian function and risk of premature menopause related to cancer treatment. *J Natl Cancer Inst Monogr* 2005; **34**: 25–7.

Sung L, Bustillo M, Mukherjee T *et al*. Sisters of women with premature ovarian failure may not be ideal ovum donors. *Fertil Steril* 1997; **67**: 912–16.

Books

National Collaborating Centre for Women's and Children's Health. *Fertility: Assessment and Treatment for People with Fertility Problems.* London: Royal College of Gynaecologists and Obstetricians Press, 2004: 126–7.

Petras K. *The Premature Menopause Book: When the 'Change of Life' comes too Early.* New York: Avon Books, 1999.

Websites

Early Menopause UK:
www.earlymenopauseuk.co.uk (last accessed 6 March 2006).
Daisy Network:
www.daisynetwork.org.uk (last accessed 6 March 2006).
International Premature Ovarian Failure Association (IPOFA):
www.pofsupport.org (last accessed 6 March 2006).
Menopause Matters:
www.menopausematters.co.uk (last accessed 6 March 2006).

13 Managing the menopause when you have other medical conditions

Gynaecological (women's) problems
Breast problems
Cardiovascular (heart and blood vessel) disease
Diabetes and thyroid disease
Neurological conditions
Gastrointestinal (gut) problems
Autoimmune diseases
Other conditions
Sources of information

Female hormones affect many body systems, so the menopause can affect other conditions, such as diabetes and migraine. Talk to your doctor if you have concerns about this. In some cases, it may be helpful to get advice from a specialist clinic. This chapter outlines the main conditions that are likely to be affected by the menopause and might affect your decision about whether or not to use hormone replacement therapy (*HRT*).

Gynaecological (women's) problems

Fibroids

Fibroids are non-cancerous growths in the muscle wall of the womb (*myometrium*). They are affected by *oestrogen* levels and often shrink after the menopause. However, they can increase in size with oestrogen, so HRT may cause heavy or painful bleeds. The effects of different types of HRT on fibroid growth are unclear, but some evidence shows that raloxifene may shrink fibroids. Your doctor may use ultrasound or a pelvic examination to assess the size of the fibroids occasionally.

Endometriosis

This describes a condition in which the tissue that lines the womb (*endometrium*) grows in the wrong places – sometimes forming cysts. It may be treated by removing the excess tissue, which sometimes may involve removing one or both ovaries (*oophorectomy*). It may also be treated by drugs that reduce oestrogen production called gonadotrophin-releasing hormone (or GnRH) analogues (eg buserelin and goserelin). In theory, HRT can reactivate the disease, even after surgery. The risks, however, seem to be small. Some gynaecologists avoid giving oestrogen alone, especially for the first six months after oophorectomy. Instead of oestrogen, they may recommend a *progestogen* on its own, continuous combined oestrogen and progestogen therapy or *tibolone* to control *vasomotor* symptoms. There is no clear evidence about which of these is best. Women who have had endometriosis may be at particular risk of the long-term effects of low oestrogen levels caused by the GnRH analogues or oophorectomy.

Cancer and abnormal growth (dysplasia) of the cervix

These are not affected by oestrogen levels, so it is safe to use HRT.

Ovarian cancer

This is not usually affected by oestrogen levels, so it is safe to use HRT. However, in certain types (called endometroid ovarian cancer), it may be safest to use oestrogen plus progestogen. Hormone therapy does not seem to increase the risk in women who carry BRCA mutations, which are linked to an increased risk of ovarian cancer.

Endometrial cancer

Use of oestrogen without progestogen carries an increased risk of endometrial cancer in women who have not had a *hysterectomy*. Therefore, HRT is usually avoided in women who have already had endometrial cancer. However, there is no evidence to show that it is dangerous, and, in fact, a small study has suggested it might even reduce the risk of a relapse. Little is known about the effects of tibolone or raloxifene after endometrial cancer.

Breast problems

Family history of breast cancer

Women with a clear family history of breast cancer should seek specialist advice about whether or not they should use HRT. This decision can be made only after the woman's personal risk of developing breast cancer has been worked out. For more information on risk factors, see Chapter 6.

Benign breast disease

Some, but by no means all, benign breast conditions carry an increased risk of breast cancer. Decisions about HRT should be made after assessing the personal risk for developing breast cancer. Only conditions that cause unusual growth (atypical *hyperplasia*) of the milk ducts or lobules are linked with an increased risk of cancer. For women with other types of benign breast conditions not linked to cancer, there is no evidence that HRT raises their risk of cancer more than it does for other women. However, HRT can cause breast pain and tenderness (mastalgia) and increase the growth of breast cysts.

Previous breast cancer

It is not clear whether or not it is safe for women who have had breast cancer to use HRT if they have menopausal symptoms. Studies have produced conflicting results. Use of tibolone is currently being studied.

Low-dose oestrogen preparations applied directly to the vagina (rather than preparations that enter the bloodstream) may be used to treat vaginal symptoms.

Women who have had breast cancer and are at high risk of *osteoporosis* (brittle bones) should seek specialist advice.

Cardiovascular (heart and blood vessel) disease

High blood pressure (hypertension)

No evidence shows that HRT, tibolone or raloxifene raise blood pressure or do any harm to women with *hypertension*. Severe hypertension is a very rare side-effect of *conjugated equine oestrogens*, but blood pressure returns to normal when treatment is stopped.

Diseases affecting the heart valves

Hormone replacement therapy can be used safely by women with valvular heart disease. Women who take *anticoagulants* (used to thin blood) sometimes have problems with irregular or heavy bleeding. This can usually be resolved by adjusting the dose of progestogen.

Raised blood lipids (hyperlipidaemia) and cholesterol

High levels of *lipids* (fats) in the blood are a risk factor for heart attacks and strokes. The most important lipids in this respect are low-density lipoprotein cholesterol (*LDL-C*), *triglyceride* and *lipoprotein a*. In contrast, high-density lipoprotein cholesterol (*HDL-C*) protects against heart disease (see Chapter 3). Different types of HRT have different effects on blood lipids (Table 13.1).

Table 13.1

Effects of hormones on lipids

Hormone	Lipid			
	HDL	LDL	Triglyceride	Lipoprotein (a)
Ideal HRT	↑↑	↓↓	↓↓	↓↓
Oral oestrogen	↑	↓↓	↑	↓↓
Transdermal oestrogen	–	↓	↓	↓
Oral progesterone derived progestogen	↑	↓	↑	↓
Oral testosterone derived progestogen	–	↓	↓	↓
Tibolone	↓	↓	↓↓	↓
Raloxifene	–	↓	–	↓

↑ Small increase
↓ Small decrease
↑↑ Big increase
↓↓ Large decrease
– No effect

If you have raised lipid levels, your doctor should tailor your HRT to your individual needs. Hormone replacement therapy can safely be taken with *statins*, which are drugs that lower levels of lipids in blood.

Deep vein clots (venous thromboembolism, VTE)

When considering HRT, your doctor will need to know if you have ever had a deep vein clot (*DVT*; sometimes called a *venous thromboembolism* or VTE) or if there is a history of these in your family.

If you have already had a VTE, you will probably be advised not to use HRT, because it can increase the risk of getting another VTE. However, in some cases, your doctor may feel that the benefits outweigh the risks. The use of oestrogen, raloxifene and *progestogens* in doses needed for HRT increases the risk of VTE, so they are probably best avoided. There are no data yet about tibolone. If you and your doctor decide that the benefits of HRT outweigh the risks, some evidence shows that gels or patches that deliver hormones through the skin might be safer than tablets.

If you have a family history of blood clots, your doctor may ask for a blood test, but a good result does not rule out the risk entirely. Some evidence shows that gels or patches that deliver hormones through the skin might be safer than tablets.

If you have had a blood clot and are currently taking long-term *warfarin* (blood-thinning treatment), you can probably use HRT as the risk of another clot is low, as long as you continue with the warfarin. However, starting warfarin treatment just so you can use HRT is not recommended, as warfarin itself carries risks, particularly of dangerous bleeding.

HRT and surgery

Although using HRT increases your risk of developing a blood clot, the risk disappears as soon as you stop the HRT. In some cases, therefore, you may be asked to stop HRT if you are planning an operation.

Diabetes and thyroid disease

Diabetes mellitus

Hormone replacement therapy seems to decrease the risk of developing diabetes and can improve the control of blood sugar in women with the condition. Diabetes affects blood lipids as well as blood sugar, but HRT, especially if delivered through the skin, seems to improve the lipid profile.

Information about the effects of HRT on *coronary* heart disease (*CHD*) is less clear. It may be good for younger postmenopausal women with diabetes, but it is not recommended for women older than 60 years or those at high risk of heart disease. Women with type 1 (early onset) diabetes are at increased risk of osteoporosis, and this may be another reason for using HRT. The effects of type 2 (adult onset) diabetes on bone mass are unclear.

Thyroid disease

An overactive *thyroid* gland (hyperthyroidism) is linked with an increased risk of osteoporosis and hip fractures. Medicines that suppress thyroid-stimulating hormone (TSH), which may be used to treat an underactive thyroid gland (hypothyroidism), may also increase the risk of osteoporosis. Women with hyperthyroidism therefore should be screened for osteoporosis. Thyroxine can be taken with HRT, but the dose may need to be increased, as oestrogen can affect the metabolism of thyroxine.

Neurological conditions

Migraine

More women than men suffer from migraine, and the headaches usually start during the teenage years and 20s. It is unusual for migraines to start after the age of 50 years. Many women with migraine get headaches around their monthly period. The menopause may be a time of increased migraine, but HRT can help, and there is no good evidence that HRT makes migraine worse.

As migraine can be triggered by changes in oestrogen levels, skin patches or vaginal rings are probably better than tablets, as they produce more stable levels of oestrogen. Too much oestrogen can trigger migraine aura (flickering lights that many people see before the headache starts), but this usually resolves if the dose is reduced. Unlike the contraceptive pill, there is no evidence that women with migraine who take HRT are at increased risk of stroke. Cyclic monthly progestogen may trigger migraine headaches in some women. Changing the type of progestogen, changing to continuous combined therapy or giving the progestogen in a patch or via an intrauterine device may solve the problem (see Chapter 4). It is safe to use migraine treatments together with HRT.

Epilepsy

There is not much information about the effects of the menopause and HRT on epilepsy. Some antiepileptic medicines may affect the way in which HRT is broken down in the liver, and herbal preparations used to treat symptoms of the menopause may interact with the antiepileptic treatment. There are no studies to show whether or not *transdermal* HRT is better than oral or whether or not women taking these medicines should take a higher dose of HRT. Some antiepileptic drugs, such as phenytoin and carbamazepine, can cause decreased bone mass and increase the risk of osteoporotic fractures.

Parkinson's disease

Population studies suggest that taking oestrogen after the menopause may reduce the risk of Parkinson's disease. The effects of HRT on women with Parkinson's disease are limited, but it seems to be safe and may even help the symptoms.

Gastrointestinal (gut) problems

Gallbladder disease

About one in 12 people in the UK older than 40 years have gallstones, and this figure rises to more than one in five of those older than 60 years. Randomized trials have shown an increased risk of gallbladder disease with oral HRT (see Chapter 8). Many doctors recommend non-oral forms of HRT (eg patches) for women with gallbladder problems, but there is little evidence to support this.

Liver disease

Most doctors recommend a non-oral route of HRT in women with liver disease, so that oestrogen enters the bloodstream directly and does not first pass through the liver. However, evidence to support this theory is limited.

Some types of liver disease, such as primary biliary cirrhosis, are linked with osteoporosis. Specialist advice may be helpful.

Crohn's disease

Women with Crohn's disease may be at increased risk of osteoporosis either from the disease itself or because of long-term treatment with *glucocorticosteroids*. Transdermal HRT is usually preferred to ensure it is absorbed properly.

Coeliac disease

Bone density is reduced in people with coeliac disease, and nearly half of all women on gluten-free diets will develop osteoporosis. This is probably caused by an inability to absorb calcium and possibly also vitamin D. Hormone replacement therapy is therefore important to reduce the risk of bone fractures. Transdermal routes may be better than oral routes.

Autoimmune diseases

Rheumatoid arthritis

This type of arthritis is caused when the body forms antibodies to tissues in the joints, which causes them to become inflamed, swell up and be painful (Figure 13.1). It is therefore different from the more common form, osteoarthritis, which is largely caused by physical wear and tear on the joints as you get older. The main symptoms are inflamed and painful joints. Women are affected about 2.5 times more often than men. Women with rheumatoid

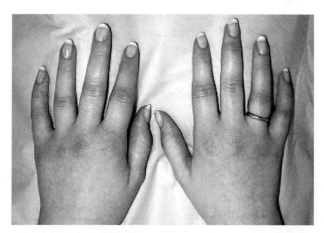

Figure 13.1 Early rheumatoid arthritis in the hands, with permission from The Arthritis Research Campaign (www.arc.org.uk and www.jointzone.org.uk)

arthritis are at increased risk of osteoporosis. This may be because of steroid treatment, lack of exercise because of stiff and painful joints and the fact that the disease itself can cause bone loss. There is no evidence that using HRT affects the risk of developing rheumatoid arthritis. In women who already have the disease, there is no evidence that HRT makes it worse. *Bisphosphonates* are also useful for reducing the risk of fractures.

Systemic lupus erythematosus

Systemic lupus erythematosus (SLE) is a rare disease of the immune system that affects many body systems, including the heart and kidneys. It usually gets worse during pregnancy, which suggests that hormone levels affect this condition. Long-term use of steroids means that women with SLE are at high risk of osteoporosis. Studies have shown that one in eight patients with SLE will have fractures, and the fracture rate for women with SLE is nearly five times higher than normal. Women with SLE should therefore benefit from anything that reduces osteoporosis. However, many doctors believe that SLE is affected by oestrogen and that HRT will increase the rate of flares. There are few studies in this area to support or disprove these ideas, so HRT should be considered with caution. Systemic lupus erythematosus may also affect blood clotting, and HRT is usually not suitable for women with a previous deep vein clot (VTE) or who have unusual blood clotting (lupus anticoagulant).

Other conditions

Asthma

Women who take HRT seem to be at slightly greater risk of developing asthma and symptoms such as wheezing. However, for most women who already have asthma, HRT does not seem to make it worse. Women who take steroid tablets (but not inhalers) for their asthma may be more likely to get osteoporosis and so may benefit from HRT.

Otosclerosis (conductive deafness)

This is an inherited condition that causes progressive deafness. The condition seems to get worse during pregnancy, and, occasionally, when affected women take the contraceptive pill. However, there is no evidence that HRT makes it worse. As the disease is naturally progressive, hearing will gradually get worse in long-term HRT users – just as it does in non-users as they get older.

Skin cancer (malignant melanoma)

This is a controversial area. Most doctors accept that there is no link between using HRT and a woman's risk of getting malignant melanoma. Studies about whether or not HRT affects the outlook for women who do get skin cancer are contradictory. This type of cancer does contain oestrogen receptors, but it is unlikely that the oestrogen in HRT increases its growth.

Age spots (dark patches on the skin) are most common in people in their 70s. They are usually found on the cheek or neck and are linked to exposure to sunlight and ultraviolet (UV) radiation. Some types of age spot (called lentigo maligna) can turn into skin cancer. Precancerous cells contain receptors for both oestrogen and *progesterone*, which suggests that levels of these hormones might affect the transformation from benign to cancerous growth.

After a transplant

Bone mass often falls after an organ or bone marrow transplant because of treatments given to prevent rejection of the transplant. Up to 80% of transplant patients will have osteoporosis (brittle bones) and up to 65% will have a fracture. Bone loss is largely due to the use of steroids (glucocorticosteroid therapy) after the transplant, but it may also be linked to immunosuppressive treatment (eg cyclosporin A or tacrolimus). There is not much information about the use of HRT in women who have received a transplant, but it should probably be considered, along with other measures to reduce osteoporosis.

Kidney (renal) failure

Patients with kidney failure (sometimes called end-stage renal disease or ESRD) are at increased risk for an early menopause, osteoporosis and heart disease. More information is needed to understand the benefits and risks of HRT and non-oestrogen alternatives for these women.

Sources of information

Journal articles

Bjoro T, Holmen J, Kruger O *et al.* Prevalence of thyroid disease, thyroid dysfunction and thyroid peroxidase antibodies in a large, unselected population. The Health Study of Nord-Trondelag (HUNT). *Eur J Endocrinol* 2000; **143**: 639–47.

Bousser MG, Conard J, Kittner S *et al.* Recommendations on the risk of ischaemic stroke associated with use of combined oral contraceptives and hormone replacement therapy in women with migraine. The International Headache Society Task Force on Combined Oral Contraceptives & Hormone Replacement Therapy. *Cephalalgia* 2000; **20**: 155–6.

Cirillo DJ, Wallace RB, Rodabough RJ *et al.* Effect of estrogen therapy on gallbladder disease. *JAMA* 2005; **293**: 330–9.

Karalis I, Beevers G, Beevers M, Lip G. Hormone replacement therapy and arterial blood pressure in postmenopausal women with hypertension. *Blood Press* 2005; **14**: 38–44.

Kwan K, Ward C, Marsden J. Is there a role for hormone replacement therapy after breast cancer? *J Br Menopause Soc* 2005; **11**: 140–4.

Lodder MC, de Jong Z, Kostense PJ *et al.* Bone mineral density in patients with rheumatoid arthritis: relation between disease severity and low bone mineral density. *Ann Rheum Dis* 2004; **63**: 1576–80.

Naldi L, Altieri A, Imberti GL *et al.* Cutaneous malignant melanoma in women. Phenotypic characteristics, sun exposure, and hormonal factors: a case–control study from Italy. *Ann Epidemiol* 2005; **15**: 545–50.

Santen RJ, Mansel R. Benign breast disorders. *N Engl J Med* 2005; **353**: 275–85.

Yee CS, Crabtree N, Skan J *et al.* Prevalence and predictors of fragility fractures in systemic lupus erythematosus. *Ann Rheum Dis* 2005; **64**: 111–13.

14 Staying healthy around and after the menopause

Looking after yourself
Information your doctor/health professional will need to know
Counselling
Sources of information

Even if you go through the menopause with few symptoms, you need to think about your long-term health. It may be helpful to talk to your doctor, nurse or health professional about this.

Most women take hormone replacement therapy (*HRT*) to reduce symptoms such as hot flushes and mood swings, but it can also have long-term benefits such as maintaining healthy bones. The following women may get special benefit from HRT:

- those who have an early menopause
- those with other risk factors for *osteoporosis* (brittle bones), such as steroid use.

You should therefore discuss the possible benefits and risks with your health professional.

If you do decide to use HRT, you need to think about how long you will take it. This is an individual decision, as the risks and benefits vary from woman to woman. You should continue with HRT as long as the benefits outweigh the potential disadvantages. There is no fixed time limit on HRT, so you need to discuss this with your doctor to work out what is best for you (see the section about how long you should take HRT in Chapter 7).

Looking after yourself

Diet and lifestyle

Healthy diet and healthy lifestyle are important throughout our lives, but the menopause may be a useful time to review your personal situation.

The huge differences in women's experience of the menopause around the world may partly be due to variations in diet (including intake of *phytoestrogens*) and lifestyle. A healthy diet and regular exercise are important in protecting against heart disease and fragile bones. Exercise may also reduce hot flushes and psychological symptoms of the menopause, such as mood swings. Weight-bearing and muscle-strengthening exercises help to maintain strong bones, but the effect is lost as soon as regular exercise stops.

Hot flushes may also be reduced by simple measures, such as avoiding getting too hot and avoiding drinks containing caffeine or alcohol.

Taking in enough calcium and vitamin D (either in foods or from supplements) is important to maintain healthy bones. Other lifestyle changes such as stopping smoking and cutting down on excess alcohol, caffeine, salt and animal proteins may help reduce bone loss and increase calcium absorption. Physical activity, stopping smoking and not being overweight will reduce the risk of cancer (see Chapter 6).

Many factors affect the risk of heart attacks and strokes. The most important are probably smoking, blood pressure and levels of *lipids* (cholesterol). Women should identify the factors that may increase their risk and identify areas of their lives that need alteration (see Chapter 6).

Cervical screening

You should continue to have cervical smears (to detect abnormalities or cancer of the womb entrance or *cervix*) every 3–5 years up to the age of about 64 years. There is no need to have them more frequently or after the age of 64 years if you are taking HRT.

Breast screening (mammography)

A mammogram is an X-ray of the breast that may detect breast cancer. In the UK, the National Health Service Breast Screening Programme uses a routine call and recall system to invite well women between the ages of 50–70 years for a screening mammogram every three years (Figure 14.1). Women older than 70 years are not routinely called for a screening mammogram, but they are entitled to request breast screening every three years. Women younger than 50 years are not offered routine screening, as mammograms seem not to be as effective in premenopausal women – possibly because the density of the breast tissue makes it more difficult to detect problems and also because the incidence of breast cancer is lower. The exception to this is women with a moderate or strong family history of breast cancer, who are eligible for a mammogram once a year between the ages of 40 and 49 years, as evidence suggests that cancer detection rates are higher in this small group of women (see Chapter 6). Ultrasound scanning of the breast is useful in assessing

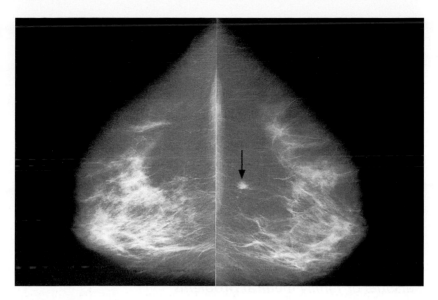

Figure 14.1 Mammogram of a normal breast on the left and of a breast with a small tumour on the right (indicated by arrow). Reproduced from Dixon (2006) with permission from Blackwell Publishing Ltd

women who have specific breast symptoms (eg a breast lump) but is not an effective screening tool.

If you have any breast symptoms of concern (such as lumps, pain or discharge), you should report them to your doctor, and a breast specialist referral may be advised.

There is no indication to have a mammogram before starting HRT, and there is no need to have screening mammograms performed more than every three years (the recommended interval between screens in the National Health Service Breast Screening Programme) for women who are taking HRT. However, if you develop any new breast symptoms, it is important that you see your doctor whether or not you are taking HRT.

Unexpected bleeding

You should tell your doctor about any unexpected change in vaginal bleeding. In such cases, your doctor may arrange for you to have some tests, such as a scan or *biopsy*, to get a small sample of the lining of the womb (*endometrium*) (see Chapter 5).

Information your doctor/health professional will need to know

Below is a checklist you can take when you see your doctor to discuss what you want to do about the menopause.

Periods, symptoms and contraception

- When was your last period?
- How frequent are/were your periods, how heavy and how long do/did they last?
- Do you get hot flushes?
- Do you get vaginal dryness?
- Do you have urinary problems?
- Have you any other symptoms?
- What contraception have you and your partner been using?

Personal or family medical problems

Tell your doctor if you know about any of the following.
- Breast cancer/ovarian cancer in close family members (parents, sisters, brothers or yourself):
  - At what age did they develop it?
- Blood clots in legs (deep vein thrombosis) or lungs (pulmonary embolism) in parents, brothers, sisters or yourself:
  - When and why? Was it after a hip or knee replacement?
  - Was the person on the 'pill' or pregnant?
  - Did they have any test to confirm the clot?
  - Were they treated with warfarin?
- Risk factors for heart disease and strokes:
  - Have you had a heart attack or stroke already?
  - Have your parents, brothers or sisters had a heart attack or stroke, and, if so, at what age?
  - Do you smoke, and, if so, how much?
  - Do you have high blood pressure or diabetes?
  - Do you have a high cholesterol level?
- Risk factors for osteoporosis (see Chapter 6 for full list):
  - Was your menopause before the age of 45?
  - Have you taken *glucocorticosteroids* for six months or more?
  - Have you ever been underweight?
  - Does osteoporosis run in your family (especially mother or sister)?
  - Have you had a fracture already, and, if so, how did it happen and where was it?

- Do you suffer from migraines (not just headaches)?
- What medicines are you taking, including herbal remedies and vitamin supplements?
- Could you be pregnant?

What do you want to do?

- Do you want to take HRT?
- If you want HRT, think about which preparation would suit you best.

Counselling

Many women feel perplexed by the changes in their body and the different treatment options available at the menopause. Getting enough information and having an understanding person to talk to are therefore very important. Your doctor, nurse or pharmacist should tell you about the benefits, risks and possible side-effects of any treatments you are being offered. Reassurance and practical advice can often reduce, or remove, some psychological aspects of the menopause. Other forms of counselling or psychotherapy may be helpful for women whose psychological symptoms are caused by a combination of changes in *oestrogen* levels and a major life event, such as bereavement or separation. Help is available from local self-help groups, bereavement counselling, Relate (marriage guidance) or assertiveness training.

Sources of information

Book

Dixon M. *ABC of Breast Diseases.* London: Blackwell Publishing Ltd, 2006.

Websites

National Electronic Library for Health:
   www.nelh.nhs.uk/ (last accessed 6 March 2006).
NHS Breast Screening Programme:
   www.cancerscreening.nhs.uk/breastscreen (last accessed 6 March 2006).
NHS Cancer Screening Programmes:
   www.cancerscreening.nhs.uk (last accessed 6 March 2006).
National Institute for Clinical Excellence:
   www.nice.org.uk (last accessed 6 March 2006).
Relate:
   www.relate.org.uk (last accessed 6 March 2006).

Word list

Note: This book uses British spellings. If you get material from the Internet, you may notice differences in American spellings. If you are searching the Internet, it is often helpful to try both the British and American spellings. In general, American doctors use 'e' instead of 'ae' and 'oe' in words such as haemorrhage and oestrogen.

Adrenals	glands around the kidneys that produce hormones
Alendronate	a bisphosphonate
Androgens	male hormones such as testosterone
Anticoagulant	a medicine that reduces blood clotting
Arrhythmia	heart rhythm problems
Artery	a type of blood vessel
Atherosclerosis	narrowing of the arteries due to 'furring up' by cholesterol
Atrophy	degeneration or wearing out of a structure
Bilateral oophorectomy	an operation to remove both ovaries
Biopsy	a sample of tissue taken for examination
Bisphosphonates	a family of medicines used to treat osteoporosis (alendronate, risedronate, ibandronate and etidronate)
Calcitonin	a medicine to treat osteoporosis
Calcitriol	a medicine to treat osteoporosis
Carcinoid syndrome	a very rare cause of hot flushes caused by tumours in the gut
Cardiovascular	relating to the heart and blood vessels
Cervix	the neck of the womb
CHD	coronary heart disease
Coagulation	the way and speed at which blood clots
Colles' fracture	type of fracture of the arm bone near the wrist
Colorectal cancer	bowel cancer

Conjugated equine oestrogens	type of HRT oestrogen sourced from horses' urine
Coronary	sometimes used as another word for a heart attack; more correctly, the name of the arteries that supply the heart with blood (coronary arteries)
Darifenacin	a medicine for urinary incontinence
Dementia	a serious progressive loss of mental function
Donepezil	a medicine for dementia
Drospirenone	a progestogen
Dual-energy X-ray absorptiometry	a way of measuring bone mineral density
Duloxetine	a medicine for urinary incontinence
DVT	deep vein thrombosis (see Venous thromboembolism)
Dydrogesterone	a progestogen
Endometrium	the lining of the uterus (womb)
Endothelia	see Endothelium
Endothelium	the inner wall of an artery (plural = *endothelia*)
Epithelium	the surface layer of cells, eg lining the vagina
Ethinyl oestradiol	a type of oestrogen usually used in the combined oral contraceptive pill
Etidronate	a bisphosphonate
Fibroids	non cancerous growths of the muscle wall of the womb
FSH	follicle-stimulating hormone (one of the female hormones produced by the pituitary gland)
Galantamine	a medicine for dementia
Glucocorticosteroid	prescribed steroids, such as hydrocortisone, prednisolone, cortisone and betamethasone
Haemorrhage	bleeding (US spelling = hemorrhage)
Haemorrhagic strokes	strokes caused by bleeding (rather than a blood clot)
HDL-C	high-density lipoprotein cholesterol – a 'good' type of cholesterol
HRT	hormone replacement therapy
Hypercholesterolaemia	raised levels of cholesterol in the blood
Hyperlipidaemia	raised levels of lipids (fats like cholesterol) in the blood
Hyperplasia	an increase in the number of cells in a tissue

Hypertension	high blood pressure
Hysterectomy	an operation to remove the womb
Hysteroscopy	a procedure to view the inside of the womb
Ibandronate	a bisphosphonate
Ischaemic stroke	stroke caused by a blood clot or blocked blood vessel
LDL-C	low-density lipoprotein cholesterol – a 'bad' type of cholesterol
Levonorgestrel	a progestogen
LH	luteinizing hormone (one of the female hormones produced by the pituitary gland)
Libido	sex drive
Lipid	fat, such as cholesterol
Lipoprotein a	a fat found in blood
Lumen	the inside of an organ, eg a blood vessel
Medroxyprogesterone acetate	a progestogen
Megestrol acetate	a progestogen
Memantine	a medicine for dementia
Menarche	the time when a girl starts having monthly periods
Milligram (mg)	one thousandth (0.001) of a gram
Microgram (μg or mcg)	one millionth (0.000001) of a gram
Myocardial infarction	heart attack
Myometrium	muscle layer or wall of the womb
Nocturia	needing to pass water at night
Oestrogen	a female sex hormone produced by the ovary (US spelling = estrogen)
Oocytes	egg cells
Oophorectomy	an operation to remove the ovaries (one or both)
Oral	taken by mouth (eg a tablet)
Osteoporosis	a condition in which the bones become very light, fragile and at risk of breaking
Ovary	female reproductive organ that produces eggs
Oxybutynin	a medicine for urinary incontinence
Parathyroid glands	small glands in the neck that produce a hormone (parathyroid hormone) that affects calcium metabolism
Parenteral	word used to describe a medicine delivered directly into the bloodstream, eg by a transdermal patch rather than orally

Phaeochromocytoma	a very rare cause of hot flushes caused by adrenal tumours
Phytoestrogens	plant oestrogens
Placebo	a dummy treatment (eg sugar pill) given as part of a clinical study to provide a comparison for the active treatment and to make sure any effects are not simply caused by patients (or doctors) thinking they are getting (or giving) a new form of treatment
Prolapse	condition in which the structures supporting organs weaken, causing them to move down in the body (eg the womb sinks into the vagina)
Progesterone	a female sex hormone produced by the ovary
Progestogens	synthetic hormones with similar effects to progesterone
Risedronate	a bisphosphonate
Rivastigmine	a medicine for dementia
Single-energy X-ray absorptiometry	a way of measuring bone mineral density
Solfenacin	a medicine for urinary incontinence
Statins	a group of drugs that lower cholesterol levels
Systemic	anything that affects the whole body
Testosterone	a male sex hormone (see androgen)
Thrombus	a blood clot
Thyroid	a gland in the neck that produces hormones such as thyroxine
Tibolone	a type of HRT
Tolterodine	a medicine for urinary incontinence
Transdermal	through the skin (eg describes an HRT patch)
Triglyceride	a blood fat
Trospium	a medicine for urinary incontinence
Urethra	the tube that carries urine out of the bladder
Uterus	womb
Vasomotor	word to describe symptoms such as hot flushes and night sweats
Venous thromboembolism	blockage of a deep vein caused by a blood clot
Warfarin	an anticoagulant

Index

Page references to *figures, tables and boxes* are shown in *italics*.
This book uses British spellings, which may differ from American spellings. See notes on pages 37 & 98.